FEARLESS & FIT

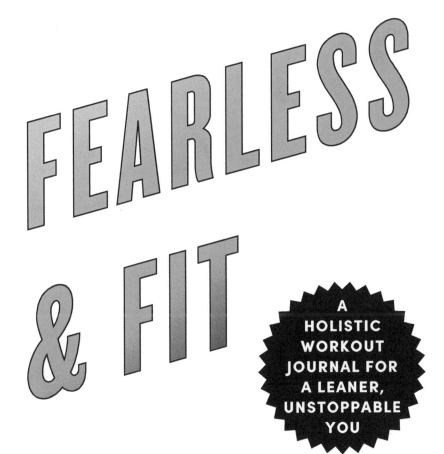

FEARLESS & FIT

A HOLISTIC WORKOUT JOURNAL FOR A LEANER, UNSTOPPABLE YOU

Illustrated by

Jesse HORA

ROCKRIDGE
PRESS

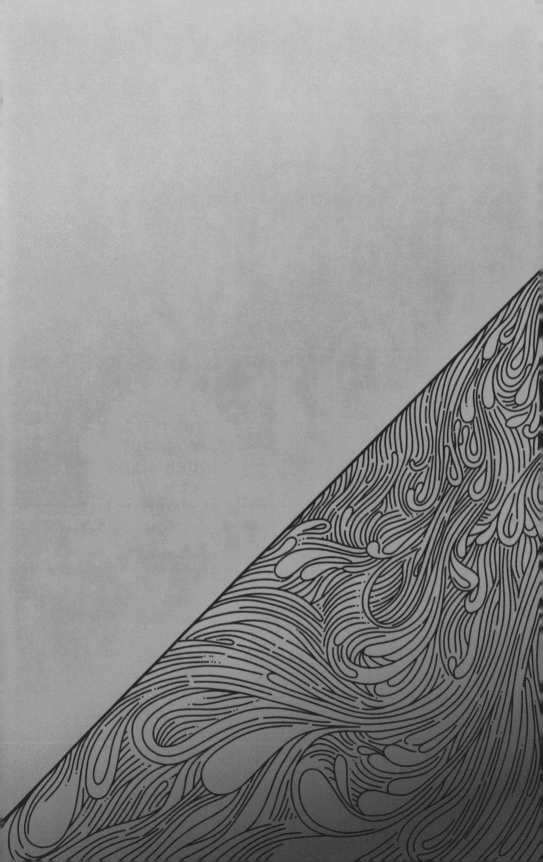

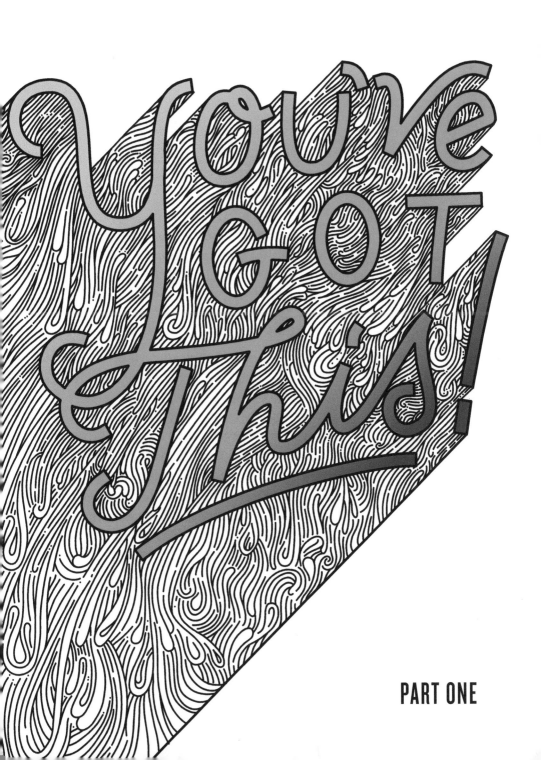

PART ONE

ALREADY AWESOME

Hey there! This is a journal for awesome women like you: women who grab life by the horns, get sh#t done, and break a sweat for noble reasons—to improve their health and boost their happiness. This journal will help you stay motivated and balanced as you begin your health journey, however big or small.

The desire to make your well-being a top priority is a sign of great wisdom and self-compassion. You'll need your body for your whole life, so taking care of it is a great (and necessary) goal, and one to congratulate yourself for.

This journal is your ally. When, where, and how often you use it is entirely up to you. You can come to this journal on good days and bad to jot down a quick note about your journey, no matter how minor. Maybe you've taken a graceful leap toward your goal, or maybe it was more of a stumble. Either way, you're still moving toward living a healthy life on your terms, which is always some-thing to celebrate. The path to progress isn't linear. Downs are just as important as ups. You've got this.

SUCCESS TIPS

Here are a few tips to help you achieve success—whatever that looks like for you.

Hydration—The importance of hydration cannot be overstated. When we exercise, our bodies lose water. If you don't replenish, you'll definitely start to feel it. Common symptoms of dehydration are low energy levels, muscle cramps, headaches, dry skin, and dizziness. Yikes! Be kind to yourself and remember to drink water before, during, and after your workout.

Rest and Recovery—Your body needs time to repair itself after a workout. Resting is just as essential as exercising when it comes to building strength, endurance, and muscle. Rest time gives your muscles and connective tissue the opportunity to rebuild themselves and come back stronger, so give them the TLC they need!

Sleep—Sleep is another important part of exercise (and of life). Consistent, quality sleep—seven to eight hours is ideal for most people—is important for your mental and physical health. What's more, the growth hormones that aid in muscle repair and reconstruction occur during REM sleep. Rest up so you're fully energized and ready to tackle the days to come.

Keep track of your water intake, schedule rest days, and create a regular sleep schedule—and hold yourself accountable for all of it. This will not only help you achieve your fitness goals, it will also help keep you happy, healthy, and balanced inside and out.

GOALS, GRIT & GRATITUDE

Before diving into your health journey, take the time to do a little self-inquiry to fuel your fitness aspirations. Pause and reflect on your noble goals. When you're ready, take a whack at the following worksheets, which will help you articulate your goals, identify your strengths, and focus on gratitude.

Got Goals?

Date: _____

My personal, exclusive, one-of-a-kind definition of healthy: _____
_____

This thing in particular inspires me to live a healthy life: _____
_____

Here's how I'm feeling in my body today: _____
_____

I sometimes worry about: _____
_____

The habit I'm kicking is: _____

The health habit I've already established is: _____

Here's where I'll be in two months: _____
_____

Here's where I'll be in six months: _____
_____

In my body, I will feel: _____
_____

In my life, I will feel: _____
_____

Notes: _____
_____
_____
_____

Inspiration

Date: _____

This person inspires me to dream: _____

This person makes me want to keep shakin' it: _____

This makes me glow: _____

A quote I love: _____

_____

Notes: _____

_____

Gratitude

Date: _____

Here's what's working for me right now in life: _____

_____

This is a quality I have that I would never change: _____

_____

A recent example of my brilliance: _____

_____

My favorite thing about my mind is: _____

_____

My favorite thing about my body is: _____

_____

This is my secret strength: _____

_____

I'm so grateful for this part of my life: _____

_____

Notes: _____

_____

_____

TALLY YOUR ASSETS

Use the following logs to track your results and measure your progress. The first log will help you capture your starting stats, and those that follow will help you track your progress. Remember, use this journal to help you tackle your fitness journey the in a way that works for you. You get to decide how and when you take stock of how it's going.

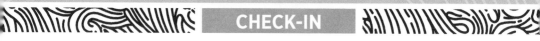

Chest: _____

Waist: _____

Hips: _____

Weight: _____

Other notes: _____

_____

_____

_____

TODAY'S THOUGHTS, FEELINGS & GOALS

_____

_____

_____

_____

_____

_____

_____

_____

_____

_____

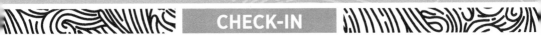

CHECK-IN

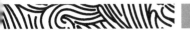

Chest: _____

Waist: _____

Hips: _____

Weight: _____

Other notes: _____

_____

_____

_____

TODAY'S THOUGHTS, FEELINGS & GOALS

_____

_____

_____

_____

_____

_____

_____

_____

_____

_____

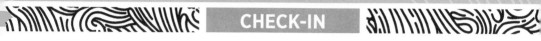

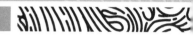

Chest: _____

Waist: _____

Hips: _____

Weight: _____

Other notes: _____

_____

_____

_____

TODAY'S THOUGHTS, FEELINGS & GOALS

_____

_____

_____

_____

_____

_____

_____

_____

_____

_____

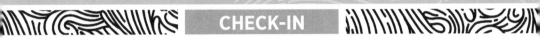
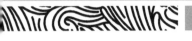

Chest: _____

Waist: _____

Hips: _____

Weight: _____

Other notes: _____

_____

_____

_____

TODAY'S THOUGHTS, FEELINGS & GOALS

_____

_____

_____

_____

_____

_____

_____

_____

_____

_____

_____

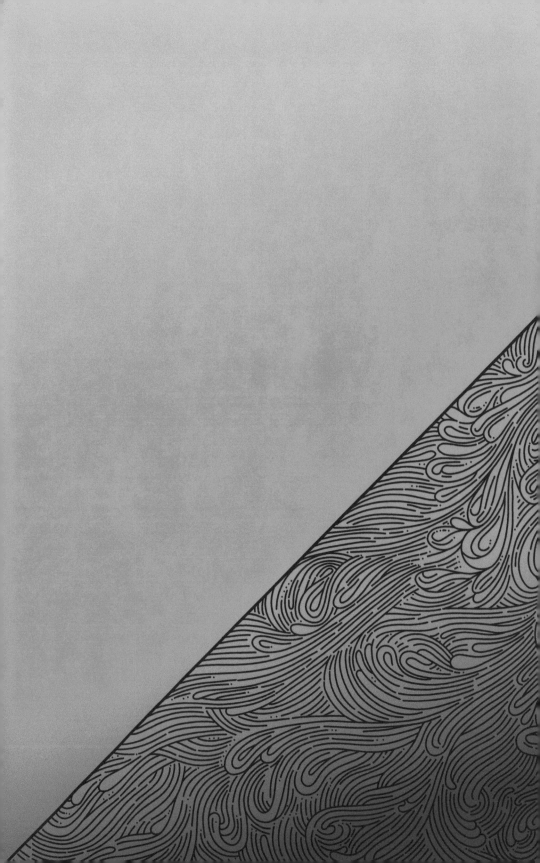

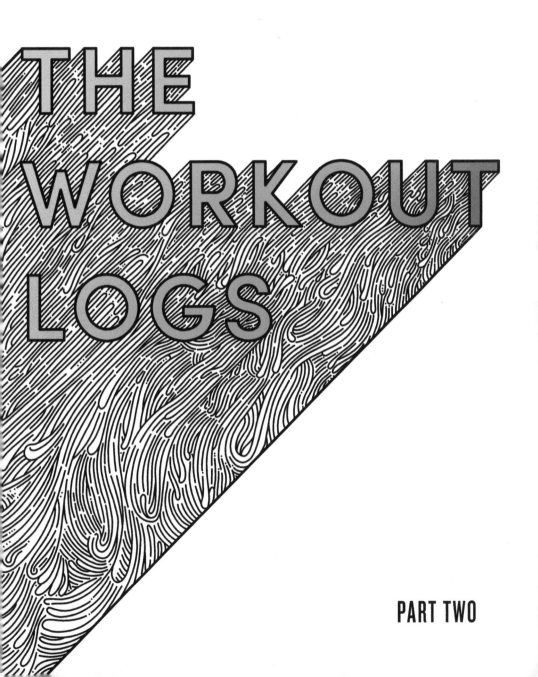

THE WORKOUT LOGS

PART TWO

WHAT'S SHAKIN'?

In this section, you can track workouts, lifestyle habits, thoughts and feelings, and anything else that feels important. You can use the notes sections to record extra details about your routine, feelings, or any other observations about your health. When you're ready, you can go back to your check-in logs to update them.

Remember, set goals that are challenging but realistic and exciting, not anxiety-inducing!

Date: _____ (S) (M) (T) (W) (Th) (F) (S)

WORKOUT

- O Cardio
- O Strength
- O Yoga
- O Other: _____

- O Pilates
- O Walk
- O Swim

- O Run
- O Bike

WORKED THESE ASSETS

- O Chest
- O Shoulders

- O Back
- O Arms

- O Legs
- O Abs

How'd it go? 😍 🙂 😐 🙁 😵

Details: _____

_____

_____

_____

_____

BONUS MOVES

- O Took the stairs
- O Added steps
- O Went for a walking meeting

- O Walked the dog
- O Went dancing with friends
- O Other: _____

MOOD & ENERGY REPORT

_____

_____

_____

_____

_____

_____

_____

STRESS LEVEL

○ Fried
○ A mixed bag
○ Could vaguely imagine being calm

○ Cucumber cool
○ I own this town

This made me smile: _____

TODAY'S MENU FEATURED

BREAKFAST
_____
_____
_____

LUNCH
_____
_____
_____

DINNER
_____
_____
_____

SNACKS
_____
_____
_____

WATER _____ OZ

My most brilliant choice today: _____

I could use a do-over on this one: _____

I'll make tomorrow even more awesome by: _____

_____

_____

Date: _____   ⓈⓂⓉⓌⓉʰⒻⓈ

WORKOUT

○ Cardio   ○ Pilates   ○ Run
○ Strength   ○ Walk   ○ Bike
○ Yoga   ○ Swim
○ Other: _____

WORKED THESE ASSETS

○ Chest   ○ Back   ○ Legs
○ Shoulders   ○ Arms   ○ Abs

How'd it go?   😍   🙂   😐   🙁   😵

Details: _____

_____

_____

_____

_____

BONUS MOVES

○ Took the stairs   ○ Walked the dog
○ Added steps   ○ Went dancing with friends
○ Went for a walking meeting ○ Other: _____

MOOD & ENERGY REPORT

_____

_____

_____

_____

_____

_____

_____

STRESS LEVEL

○ Fried
○ A mixed bag
○ Could vaguely imagine being calm

○ Cucumber cool
○ I own this town

This made me smile: _____

TODAY'S MENU FEATURED

BREAKFAST
_____
_____
_____

LUNCH
_____
_____
_____

DINNER
_____
_____
_____

SNACKS
_____
_____
_____

WATER _____ OZ

My most brilliant choice today: _____
I could use a do-over on this one: _____
I'll make tomorrow even more awesome by: _____
_____
_____

Date: _____   (S) (M) (T) (W) (Th) (F) (S)

WORKOUT

- ◯ Cardio
- ◯ Strength
- ◯ Yoga
- ◯ Other: _____

- ◯ Pilates
- ◯ Walk
- ◯ Swim

- ◯ Run
- ◯ Bike

WORKED THESE ASSETS

- ◯ Chest
- ◯ Shoulders

- ◯ Back
- ◯ Arms

- ◯ Legs
- ◯ Abs

How'd it go? 😍 🙂 😐 🙁 😵

Details: _____
_____
_____
_____
_____

BONUS MOVES

- ◯ Took the stairs
- ◯ Added steps
- ◯ Went for a walking meeting

- ◯ Walked the dog
- ◯ Went dancing with friends
- ◯ Other: _____

MOOD & ENERGY REPORT

_____
_____
_____
_____
_____
_____
_____

○ Fried   ○ Cucumber cool
○ A mixed bag   ○ I own this town
○ Could vaguely imagine
  being calm

This made me smile: _____

TODAY'S MENU FEATURED

BREAKFAST
_____
_____
_____

LUNCH
_____
_____
_____

DINNER
_____
_____
_____

SNACKS
_____
_____
_____

WATER _____ OZ

My most brilliant choice today: _____

I could use a do-over on this one: _____

I'll make tomorrow even more awesome by: _____

_____

_____

Date: _____ （S）（M）（T）（W）（Th）（F）（S）

WORKOUT

- ◯ Cardio
- ◯ Strength
- ◯ Yoga
- ◯ Other: _____

- ◯ Pilates
- ◯ Walk
- ◯ Swim

- ◯ Run
- ◯ Bike

WORKED THESE ASSETS

- ◯ Chest
- ◯ Shoulders

- ◯ Back
- ◯ Arms

- ◯ Legs
- ◯ Abs

How'd it go?   😍   🙂   😐   🙁   😵

Details: _____
_____
_____
_____
_____

BONUS MOVES

- ◯ Took the stairs
- ◯ Added steps
- ◯ Went for a walking meeting

- ◯ Walked the dog
- ◯ Went dancing with friends
- ◯ Other: _____

MOOD & ENERGY REPORT

_____
_____
_____
_____
_____
_____
_____

STRESS LEVEL

○ Fried
○ A mixed bag
○ Could vaguely imagine being calm

○ Cucumber cool
○ I own this town

This made me smile: _____

TODAY'S MENU FEATURED

BREAKFAST
_____
_____
_____

LUNCH
_____
_____
_____

DINNER
_____
_____
_____

SNACKS
_____
_____
_____

WATER _____ OZ

My most brilliant choice today: _____

I could use a do-over on this one: _____

I'll make tomorrow even more awesome by: _____

_____

_____

Date: _____ (S) (M) (T) (W) (Th) (F) (S)

WORKOUT

- ◯ Cardio
- ◯ Strength
- ◯ Yoga
- ◯ Other: _____

- ◯ Pilates
- ◯ Walk
- ◯ Swim

- ◯ Run
- ◯ Bike

WORKED THESE ASSETS

- ◯ Chest
- ◯ Shoulders

- ◯ Back
- ◯ Arms

- ◯ Legs
- ◯ Abs

How'd it go?   😍   🙂   😐   🙁   😵

Details: _____

_____

_____

_____

_____

BONUS MOVES

- ◯ Took the stairs
- ◯ Added steps
- ◯ Went for a walking meeting

- ◯ Walked the dog
- ◯ Went dancing with friends
- ◯ Other: _____

MOOD & ENERGY REPORT

_____

_____

_____

_____

_____

_____

_____

○ Fried
○ A mixed bag
○ Could vaguely imagine
   being calm

○ Cucumber cool
○ I own this town

This made me smile: _____

TODAY'S MENU FEATURED

BREAKFAST
_____
_____
_____

LUNCH
_____
_____
_____

DINNER
_____
_____
_____

SNACKS
_____
_____
_____

WATER _____ OZ

My most brilliant choice today: _____

I could use a do-over on this one: _____

I'll make tomorrow even more awesome by: _____

_____

_____

Date: _____   (S) (M) (T) (W) (Th) (F) (S)

WORKOUT

○ Cardio   ○ Pilates   ○ Run
○ Strength   ○ Walk   ○ Bike
○ Yoga   ○ Swim
○ Other: _____

WORKED THESE ASSETS

○ Chest   ○ Back   ○ Legs
○ Shoulders   ○ Arms   ○ Abs

How'd it go?   (☺)   (☺)   (☺)   (☹)   (☹)

Details: _____
_____
_____
_____
_____

BONUS MOVES

○ Took the stairs   ○ Walked the dog
○ Added steps   ○ Went dancing with friends
○ Went for a walking meeting ○ Other: _____

MOOD & ENERGY REPORT

_____
_____
_____
_____
_____
_____
_____

○ Fried
○ A mixed bag
○ Could vaguely imagine being calm

○ Cucumber cool
○ I own this town

This made me smile: _____

TODAY'S MENU FEATURED

BREAKFAST
_____
_____
_____

LUNCH
_____
_____
_____

DINNER
_____
_____
_____

SNACKS
_____
_____
_____

WATER _____ OZ

My most brilliant choice today: _____

I could use a do-over on this one: _____

I'll make tomorrow even more awesome by: _____

_____

_____

Date: _____   (S) (M) (T) (W) (Th) (F) (S)

WORKOUT

- ◯ Cardio
- ◯ Strength
- ◯ Yoga
- ◯ Other: _____

- ◯ Pilates
- ◯ Walk
- ◯ Swim

- ◯ Run
- ◯ Bike

WORKED THESE ASSETS

- ◯ Chest
- ◯ Shoulders

- ◯ Back
- ◯ Arms

- ◯ Legs
- ◯ Abs

How'd it go?   😍   🙂   😐   🙁   😵

Details: _____
_____
_____
_____
_____

BONUS MOVES

- ◯ Took the stairs
- ◯ Added steps
- ◯ Went for a walking meeting

- ◯ Walked the dog
- ◯ Went dancing with friends
- ◯ Other: _____

MOOD & ENERGY REPORT

_____
_____
_____
_____
_____
_____
_____

STRESS LEVEL

◯ Fried
◯ A mixed bag
◯ Could vaguely imagine being calm

◯ Cucumber cool
◯ I own this town

This made me smile: _____

TODAY'S MENU FEATURED

BREAKFAST
_____
_____
_____

LUNCH
_____
_____
_____

DINNER
_____
_____
_____

SNACKS
_____
_____
_____

WATER _____ OZ

My most brilliant choice today: _____

I could use a do-over on this one: _____

I'll make tomorrow even more awesome by: _____

_____

_____

Date: _____ Ⓢ Ⓜ Ⓣ Ⓦ (Th) Ⓕ Ⓢ

WORKOUT

○ Cardio   ○ Pilates   ○ Run
○ Strength   ○ Walk   ○ Bike
○ Yoga   ○ Swim
○ Other: _____

WORKED THESE ASSETS

○ Chest   ○ Back   ○ Legs
○ Shoulders   ○ Arms   ○ Abs

How'd it go?   😍   🙂   😐   🙁   😵

Details: _____
_____
_____
_____
_____

BONUS MOVES

○ Took the stairs   ○ Walked the dog
○ Added steps   ○ Went dancing with friends
○ Went for a walking meeting   ○ Other: _____

MOOD & ENERGY REPORT

_____
_____
_____
_____
_____
_____
_____

STRESS LEVEL

- ◯ Fried
- ◯ A mixed bag
- ◯ Could vaguely imagine being calm
- ◯ Cucumber cool
- ◯ I own this town

This made me smile: _____

TODAY'S MENU FEATURED

BREAKFAST
_____
_____
_____

LUNCH
_____
_____
_____

DINNER
_____
_____
_____

SNACKS
_____
_____
_____

WATER _____ OZ

My most brilliant choice today: _____

I could use a do-over on this one: _____

I'll make tomorrow even more awesome by: _____
_____
_____

Date: _____ ⓈⓂⓉⓌ(Th)ⒻⓈ

WORKOUT

- ◯ Cardio
- ◯ Strength
- ◯ Yoga
- ◯ Other: _____

- ◯ Pilates
- ◯ Walk
- ◯ Swim

- ◯ Run
- ◯ Bike

WORKED THESE ASSETS

- ◯ Chest
- ◯ Shoulders

- ◯ Back
- ◯ Arms

- ◯ Legs
- ◯ Abs

How'd it go? 😍 🙂 😐 🙁 😵

Details: _____

_____

_____

_____

_____

BONUS MOVES

- ◯ Took the stairs
- ◯ Added steps
- ◯ Went for a walking meeting

- ◯ Walked the dog
- ◯ Went dancing with friends
- ◯ Other: _____

MOOD & ENERGY REPORT

_____

_____

_____

_____

_____

_____

_____

STRESS LEVEL

◯ Fried
◯ A mixed bag
◯ Could vaguely imagine
   being calm

◯ Cucumber cool
◯ I own this town

This made me smile: _____

TODAY'S MENU FEATURED

BREAKFAST
_____
_____
_____

LUNCH
_____
_____
_____

DINNER
_____
_____
_____

SNACKS
_____
_____
_____

WATER _____ OZ

My most brilliant choice today: _____

I could use a do-over on this one: _____

I'll make tomorrow even more awesome by: _____

_____

_____

Date: _____ (S) (M) (T) (W) (Th) (F) (S)

WORKOUT

- ○ Cardio
- ○ Strength
- ○ Yoga
- ○ Other: _____

- ○ Pilates
- ○ Walk
- ○ Swim

- ○ Run
- ○ Bike

WORKED THESE ASSETS

- ○ Chest
- ○ Shoulders

- ○ Back
- ○ Arms

- ○ Legs
- ○ Abs

How'd it go?   (☺)   (☺)   (😐)   (🙁)   (😵)

Details: _____

_____

_____

_____

_____

BONUS MOVES

- ○ Took the stairs
- ○ Added steps
- ○ Went for a walking meeting

- ○ Walked the dog
- ○ Went dancing with friends
- ○ Other: _____

MOOD & ENERGY REPORT

_____

_____

_____

_____

_____

_____

_____

STRESS LEVEL

◯ Fried
◯ A mixed bag
◯ Could vaguely imagine being calm

◯ Cucumber cool
◯ I own this town

This made me smile: _____

TODAY'S MENU FEATURED

BREAKFAST
_____
_____
_____

LUNCH
_____
_____
_____

DINNER
_____
_____
_____

SNACKS
_____
_____
_____

WATER _____ OZ

My most brilliant choice today: _____

I could use a do-over on this one: _____

I'll make tomorrow even more awesome by: _____

_____

_____

Date: _____   (S) (M) (T) (W) (Th) (F) (S)

WORKOUT

- ◯ Cardio
- ◯ Strength
- ◯ Yoga
- ◯ Other: _____

- ◯ Pilates
- ◯ Walk
- ◯ Swim

- ◯ Run
- ◯ Bike

WORKED THESE ASSETS

- ◯ Chest
- ◯ Shoulders

- ◯ Back
- ◯ Arms

- ◯ Legs
- ◯ Abs

How'd it go?   😍   😊   😐   🙁   😵

Details: _____

_____

_____

_____

_____

BONUS MOVES

- ◯ Took the stairs
- ◯ Added steps
- ◯ Went for a walking meeting

- ◯ Walked the dog
- ◯ Went dancing with friends
- ◯ Other: _____

MOOD & ENERGY REPORT

_____

_____

_____

_____

_____

_____

◯ Fried
◯ A mixed bag
◯ Could vaguely imagine
   being calm

◯ Cucumber cool
◯ I own this town

This made me smile: _____

TODAY'S MENU FEATURED

BREAKFAST
_____
_____
_____

LUNCH
_____
_____
_____

DINNER
_____
_____
_____

SNACKS
_____
_____
_____

WATER _____ OZ

My most brilliant choice today: _____

I could use a do-over on this one: _____

I'll make tomorrow even more awesome by: _____

_____

_____

Date: _____ (S) (M) (T) (W) (Th) (F) (S)

WORKOUT

- ◯ Cardio
- ◯ Strength
- ◯ Yoga
- ◯ Other: _____

- ◯ Pilates
- ◯ Walk
- ◯ Swim

- ◯ Run
- ◯ Bike

WORKED THESE ASSETS

- ◯ Chest
- ◯ Shoulders

- ◯ Back
- ◯ Arms

- ◯ Legs
- ◯ Abs

How'd it go?   😍   🙂   😐   🙁   😵

Details: _____
_____
_____
_____
_____

BONUS MOVES

- ◯ Took the stairs
- ◯ Added steps
- ◯ Went for a walking meeting

- ◯ Walked the dog
- ◯ Went dancing with friends
- ◯ Other: _____

MOOD & ENERGY REPORT

_____
_____
_____
_____
_____
_____
_____

STRESS LEVEL

○ Fried
○ A mixed bag
○ Could vaguely imagine being calm

○ Cucumber cool
○ I own this town

This made me smile: _____

TODAY'S MENU FEATURED

BREAKFAST
_____
_____
_____

LUNCH
_____
_____
_____

DINNER
_____
_____
_____

SNACKS
_____
_____
_____

WATER _____ OZ

My most brilliant choice today: _____

I could use a do-over on this one: _____

I'll make tomorrow even more awesome by: _____

_____
_____

Date: _____   (S) (M) (T) (W) (Th) (F) (S)

WORKOUT

○ Cardio   ○ Pilates   ○ Run
○ Strength   ○ Walk   ○ Bike
○ Yoga   ○ Swim
○ Other: _____

WORKED THESE ASSETS

○ Chest   ○ Back   ○ Legs
○ Shoulders   ○ Arms   ○ Abs

How'd it go?   😍   🙂   😐   🙁   😵

Details: _____
_____
_____
_____
_____

BONUS MOVES

○ Took the stairs   ○ Walked the dog
○ Added steps   ○ Went dancing with friends
○ Went for a walking meeting   ○ Other: _____

MOOD & ENERGY REPORT

_____
_____
_____
_____
_____
_____
_____

○ Fried   ○ Cucumber cool
○ A mixed bag   ○ I own this town
○ Could vaguely imagine
   being calm

This made me smile: _____

TODAY'S MENU FEATURED

BREAKFAST
_____
_____
_____

LUNCH
_____
_____
_____

DINNER
_____
_____
_____

SNACKS
_____
_____
_____

WATER _____ OZ

My most brilliant choice today: _____

I could use a do-over on this one: _____

I'll make tomorrow even more awesome by: _____

_____

_____

Date: _____   (S) (M) (T) (W) (Th) (F) (S)

WORKOUT

- ◯ Cardio   ◯ Pilates   ◯ Run
- ◯ Strength   ◯ Walk   ◯ Bike
- ◯ Yoga   ◯ Swim
- ◯ Other: _____

WORKED THESE ASSETS

- ◯ Chest   ◯ Back   ◯ Legs
- ◯ Shoulders   ◯ Arms   ◯ Abs

How'd it go?   😍   🙂   😐   🙁   😵

Details: _____
_____
_____
_____
_____

BONUS MOVES

- ◯ Took the stairs   ◯ Walked the dog
- ◯ Added steps   ◯ Went dancing with friends
- ◯ Went for a walking meeting   ◯ Other: _____

MOOD & ENERGY REPORT

_____
_____
_____
_____
_____
_____

STRESS LEVEL

○ Fried
○ A mixed bag
○ Could vaguely imagine
   being calm

○ Cucumber cool
○ I own this town

This made me smile: _____

TODAY'S MENU FEATURED

BREAKFAST
_____
_____
_____

LUNCH
_____
_____
_____

DINNER
_____
_____
_____

SNACKS
_____
_____
_____

WATER _____ OZ

My most brilliant choice today: _____

I could use a do-over on this one: _____

I'll make tomorrow even more awesome by: _____

_____
_____

Date: _____ (S) (M) (T) (W) (Th) (F) (S)

WORKOUT

- ◯ Cardio
- ◯ Strength
- ◯ Yoga
- ◯ Other: _____

- ◯ Pilates
- ◯ Walk
- ◯ Swim

- ◯ Run
- ◯ Bike

WORKED THESE ASSETS

- ◯ Chest
- ◯ Shoulders

- ◯ Back
- ◯ Arms

- ◯ Legs
- ◯ Abs

How'd it go?   😍   🙂   😐   🙁   😵

Details: _____

_____

_____

_____

_____

BONUS MOVES

- ◯ Took the stairs
- ◯ Added steps
- ◯ Went for a walking meeting

- ◯ Walked the dog
- ◯ Went dancing with friends
- ◯ Other: _____

MOOD & ENERGY REPORT

_____

_____

_____

_____

_____

_____

_____

STRESS LEVEL

○ Fried
○ A mixed bag
○ Could vaguely imagine being calm

○ Cucumber cool
○ I own this town

This made me smile: _____

TODAY'S MENU FEATURED

BREAKFAST
_____
_____
_____

LUNCH
_____
_____
_____

DINNER
_____
_____
_____

SNACKS
_____
_____
_____

WATER _____ OZ

My most brilliant choice today: _____

I could use a do-over on this one: _____

I'll make tomorrow even more awesome by: _____

_____

_____

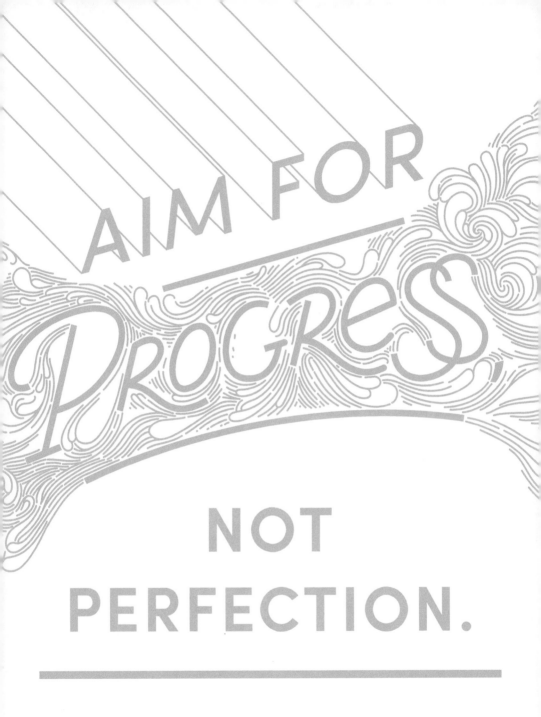

AIM FOR Progress

NOT PERFECTION.

Date: _____ (S) (M) (T) (W) (Th) (F) (S)

WORKOUT

- ○ Cardio
- ○ Strength
- ○ Yoga
- ○ Other: _____

- ○ Pilates
- ○ Walk
- ○ Swim

- ○ Run
- ○ Bike

WORKED THESE ASSETS

- ○ Chest
- ○ Shoulders

- ○ Back
- ○ Arms

- ○ Legs
- ○ Abs

How'd it go?   😍   🙂   😐   🙁   😵

Details: _____

_____

_____

_____

_____

BONUS MOVES

- ○ Took the stairs
- ○ Added steps
- ○ Went for a walking meeting

- ○ Walked the dog
- ○ Went dancing with friends
- ○ Other: _____

MOOD & ENERGY REPORT

_____

_____

_____

_____

_____

_____

_____

STRESS LEVEL

○ Fried
○ A mixed bag
○ Could vaguely imagine being calm

○ Cucumber cool
○ I own this town

This made me smile: _____

TODAY'S MENU FEATURED

BREAKFAST
_____
_____
_____

LUNCH
_____
_____
_____

DINNER
_____
_____
_____

SNACKS
_____
_____
_____

WATER _____ OZ

My most brilliant choice today: _____

I could use a do-over on this one: _____

I'll make tomorrow even more awesome by: _____

_____

_____

Date: _____ (S) (M) (T) (W) (Th) (F) (S)

WORKOUT

- ◯ Cardio
- ◯ Strength
- ◯ Yoga
- ◯ Other: _____

- ◯ Pilates
- ◯ Walk
- ◯ Swim

- ◯ Run
- ◯ Bike

WORKED THESE ASSETS

- ◯ Chest
- ◯ Shoulders

- ◯ Back
- ◯ Arms

- ◯ Legs
- ◯ Abs

How'd it go?   😍   🙂   😐   🙁   😵

Details: _____

_____

_____

_____

_____

BONUS MOVES

- ◯ Took the stairs
- ◯ Added steps
- ◯ Went for a walking meeting

- ◯ Walked the dog
- ◯ Went dancing with friends
- ◯ Other: _____

MOOD & ENERGY REPORT

_____

_____

_____

_____

_____

_____

_____

STRESS LEVEL

- ◯ Fried
- ◯ A mixed bag
- ◯ Could vaguely imagine being calm

- ◯ Cucumber cool
- ◯ I own this town

This made me smile: _____

TODAY'S MENU FEATURED

BREAKFAST
_____
_____
_____

LUNCH
_____
_____
_____

DINNER
_____
_____
_____

SNACKS
_____
_____
_____

WATER _____ OZ

My most brilliant choice today: _____

I could use a do-over on this one: _____

I'll make tomorrow even more awesome by: _____

_____
_____

Date: _____ (S) (M) (T) (W) (Th) (F) (S)

WORKOUT

- ( ) Cardio
- ( ) Strength
- ( ) Yoga
- ( ) Other: _____

- ( ) Pilates
- ( ) Walk
- ( ) Swim

- ( ) Run
- ( ) Bike

WORKED THESE ASSETS

- ( ) Chest
- ( ) Shoulders

- ( ) Back
- ( ) Arms

- ( ) Legs
- ( ) Abs

How'd it go?   (◕‿◕)   (◠‿◠)   (◠_◠)   (◠︵◠)   (×_×)

Details: _____

_____

_____

_____

_____

BONUS MOVES

- ( ) Took the stairs
- ( ) Added steps
- ( ) Went for a walking meeting

- ( ) Walked the dog
- ( ) Went dancing with friends
- ( ) Other: _____

MOOD & ENERGY REPORT

_____

_____

_____

_____

_____

_____

_____

◯ Fried
◯ A mixed bag
◯ Could vaguely imagine being calm

◯ Cucumber cool
◯ I own this town

This made me smile: _____

TODAY'S MENU FEATURED

BREAKFAST
_____
_____
_____

LUNCH
_____
_____
_____

DINNER
_____
_____
_____

SNACKS
_____
_____
_____

WATER _____ OZ

My most brilliant choice today: _____

I could use a do-over on this one: _____

I'll make tomorrow even more awesome by: _____

_____

_____

Date: _____ (S) (M) (T) (W) (Th) (F) (S)

WORKOUT

- ◯ Cardio
- ◯ Strength
- ◯ Yoga
- ◯ Other: _____

- ◯ Pilates
- ◯ Walk
- ◯ Swim

- ◯ Run
- ◯ Bike

WORKED THESE ASSETS

- ◯ Chest
- ◯ Shoulders

- ◯ Back
- ◯ Arms

- ◯ Legs
- ◯ Abs

How'd it go? 😍 🙂 😐 🙁 😵

Details: _____

_____

_____

_____

_____

BONUS MOVES

- ◯ Took the stairs
- ◯ Added steps
- ◯ Went for a walking meeting

- ◯ Walked the dog
- ◯ Went dancing with friends
- ◯ Other: _____

MOOD & ENERGY REPORT

_____

_____

_____

_____

_____

_____

_____

STRESS LEVEL

○ Fried
○ A mixed bag
○ Could vaguely imagine being calm

○ Cucumber cool
○ I own this town

This made me smile: _____

TODAY'S MENU FEATURED

BREAKFAST
_____
_____
_____

LUNCH
_____
_____
_____

DINNER
_____
_____
_____

SNACKS
_____
_____
_____

WATER _____ OZ

My most brilliant choice today: _____

I could use a do-over on this one: _____

I'll make tomorrow even more awesome by: _____

_____

_____

Date: _____ S M T W Th F S

WORKOUT

- ◯ Cardio
- ◯ Strength
- ◯ Yoga
- ◯ Other: _____

- ◯ Pilates
- ◯ Walk
- ◯ Swim

- ◯ Run
- ◯ Bike

WORKED THESE ASSETS

- ◯ Chest
- ◯ Shoulders

- ◯ Back
- ◯ Arms

- ◯ Legs
- ◯ Abs

How'd it go? 😍 🙂 😐 🙁 😵

Details: _____

_____

_____

_____

_____

BONUS MOVES

- ◯ Took the stairs
- ◯ Added steps
- ◯ Went for a walking meeting

- ◯ Walked the dog
- ◯ Went dancing with friends
- ◯ Other: _____

MOOD & ENERGY REPORT

_____

_____

_____

_____

_____

_____

_____

STRESS LEVEL

○ Fried
○ A mixed bag
○ Could vaguely imagine being calm

○ Cucumber cool
○ I own this town

This made me smile: _____

TODAY'S MENU FEATURED

BREAKFAST
_____
_____
_____

LUNCH
_____
_____
_____

DINNER
_____
_____
_____

SNACKS
_____
_____
_____

WATER _____ OZ

My most brilliant choice today: _____

I could use a do-over on this one: _____

I'll make tomorrow even more awesome by: _____

_____
_____

Date: _____   (S) (M) (T) (W) (Th) (F) (S)

WORKOUT

- ◯ Cardio
- ◯ Strength
- ◯ Yoga
- ◯ Other: _____

- ◯ Pilates
- ◯ Walk
- ◯ Swim

- ◯ Run
- ◯ Bike

WORKED THESE ASSETS

- ◯ Chest
- ◯ Shoulders

- ◯ Back
- ◯ Arms

- ◯ Legs
- ◯ Abs

How'd it go?   😍   😊   😐   🙁   😵

Details: _____
_____
_____
_____
_____

BONUS MOVES

- ◯ Took the stairs
- ◯ Added steps
- ◯ Went for a walking meeting

- ◯ Walked the dog
- ◯ Went dancing with friends
- ◯ Other: _____

MOOD & ENERGY REPORT

_____
_____
_____
_____
_____
_____
_____

STRESS LEVEL

◯ Fried
◯ A mixed bag
◯ Could vaguely imagine being calm

◯ Cucumber cool
◯ I own this town

This made me smile: _____

TODAY'S MENU FEATURED

BREAKFAST
_____
_____
_____

LUNCH
_____
_____
_____

DINNER
_____
_____
_____

SNACKS
_____
_____
_____

WATER _____ OZ

My most brilliant choice today: _____

I could use a do-over on this one: _____

I'll make tomorrow even more awesome by: _____

_____
_____

Date: _____   (S) (M) (T) (W) (Th) (F) (S)

WORKOUT

- ◯ Cardio
- ◯ Strength
- ◯ Yoga
- ◯ Other: _____

- ◯ Pilates
- ◯ Walk
- ◯ Swim

- ◯ Run
- ◯ Bike

WORKED THESE ASSETS

- ◯ Chest
- ◯ Shoulders

- ◯ Back
- ◯ Arms

- ◯ Legs
- ◯ Abs

How'd it go?   😍   🙂   😐   🙁   😵

Details: _____

_____

_____

_____

_____

BONUS MOVES

- ◯ Took the stairs
- ◯ Added steps
- ◯ Went for a walking meeting

- ◯ Walked the dog
- ◯ Went dancing with friends
- ◯ Other: _____

MOOD & ENERGY REPORT

_____

_____

_____

_____

_____

_____

_____

STRESS LEVEL

○ Fried
○ A mixed bag
○ Could vaguely imagine being calm

○ Cucumber cool
○ I own this town

This made me smile: _____

TODAY'S MENU FEATURED

BREAKFAST
_____
_____
_____

LUNCH
_____
_____
_____

DINNER
_____
_____
_____

SNACKS
_____
_____
_____

WATER _____ OZ

My most brilliant choice today: _____

I could use a do-over on this one: _____

I'll make tomorrow even more awesome by: _____

_____
_____

Date: _____   (S) (M) (T) (W) (Th) (F) (S)

WORKOUT

- ◯ Cardio
- ◯ Strength
- ◯ Yoga
- ◯ Other: _____

- ◯ Pilates
- ◯ Walk
- ◯ Swim

- ◯ Run
- ◯ Bike

WORKED THESE ASSETS

- ◯ Chest
- ◯ Shoulders

- ◯ Back
- ◯ Arms

- ◯ Legs
- ◯ Abs

How'd it go?   😍   🙂   😐   🙁   😵

Details: _____
_____
_____
_____
_____

BONUS MOVES

- ◯ Took the stairs
- ◯ Added steps
- ◯ Went for a walking meeting

- ◯ Walked the dog
- ◯ Went dancing with friends
- ◯ Other: _____

MOOD & ENERGY REPORT

_____
_____
_____
_____
_____
_____
_____

○ Fried
○ A mixed bag
○ Could vaguely imagine being calm

○ Cucumber cool
○ I own this town

This made me smile: _____

TODAY'S MENU FEATURED

BREAKFAST
_____
_____
_____

LUNCH
_____
_____
_____

DINNER
_____
_____
_____

SNACKS
_____
_____
_____

WATER _____ OZ

My most brilliant choice today: _____

I could use a do-over on this one: _____

I'll make tomorrow even more awesome by: _____

_____

_____

Date: _____ (S) (M) (T) (W) (Th) (F) (S)

WORKOUT

- ◯ Cardio
- ◯ Strength
- ◯ Yoga
- ◯ Other: _____

- ◯ Pilates
- ◯ Walk
- ◯ Swim

- ◯ Run
- ◯ Bike

WORKED THESE ASSETS

- ◯ Chest
- ◯ Shoulders

- ◯ Back
- ◯ Arms

- ◯ Legs
- ◯ Abs

How'd it go?   😍   🙂   😐   🙁   😵

Details: _____

_____

_____

_____

_____

BONUS MOVES

- ◯ Took the stairs
- ◯ Added steps
- ◯ Went for a walking meeting

- ◯ Walked the dog
- ◯ Went dancing with friends
- ◯ Other: _____

MOOD & ENERGY REPORT

_____

_____

_____

_____

_____

_____

_____

STRESS LEVEL

○ Fried
○ A mixed bag
○ Could vaguely imagine being calm

○ Cucumber cool
○ I own this town

This made me smile: _____

TODAY'S MENU FEATURED

BREAKFAST
_____
_____
_____

LUNCH
_____
_____
_____

DINNER
_____
_____
_____

SNACKS
_____
_____
_____

WATER _____ OZ

My most brilliant choice today: _____

I could use a do-over on this one: _____

I'll make tomorrow even more awesome by: _____

_____

_____

Date: _____   (S) (M) (T) (W) (Th) (F) (S)

WORKOUT

- ◯ Cardio
- ◯ Strength
- ◯ Yoga
- ◯ Other: _____

- ◯ Pilates
- ◯ Walk
- ◯ Swim

- ◯ Run
- ◯ Bike

WORKED THESE ASSETS

- ◯ Chest
- ◯ Shoulders

- ◯ Back
- ◯ Arms

- ◯ Legs
- ◯ Abs

How'd it go?   😍   🙂   😐   🙁   😵

Details: _____

_____

_____

_____

_____

BONUS MOVES

- ◯ Took the stairs
- ◯ Added steps
- ◯ Went for a walking meeting

- ◯ Walked the dog
- ◯ Went dancing with friends
- ◯ Other: _____

MOOD & ENERGY REPORT

_____

_____

_____

_____

_____

_____

_____

○ Fried
○ A mixed bag
○ Could vaguely imagine being calm

○ Cucumber cool
○ I own this town

This made me smile: _____

TODAY'S MENU FEATURED

BREAKFAST
_____
_____
_____

LUNCH
_____
_____
_____

DINNER
_____
_____
_____

SNACKS
_____
_____
_____

WATER _____ OZ

My most brilliant choice today: _____

I could use a do-over on this one: _____

I'll make tomorrow even more awesome by: _____

_____

_____

Date: _____   (S) (M) (T) (W) (Th) (F) (S)

WORKOUT

- ◯ Cardio
- ◯ Strength
- ◯ Yoga
- ◯ Other: _____

- ◯ Pilates
- ◯ Walk
- ◯ Swim

- ◯ Run
- ◯ Bike

WORKED THESE ASSETS

- ◯ Chest
- ◯ Shoulders

- ◯ Back
- ◯ Arms

- ◯ Legs
- ◯ Abs

How'd it go?   😍   🙂   😐   🙁   😵

Details: _____

_____

_____

_____

_____

BONUS MOVES

- ◯ Took the stairs
- ◯ Added steps
- ◯ Went for a walking meeting

- ◯ Walked the dog
- ◯ Went dancing with friends
- ◯ Other: _____

MOOD & ENERGY REPORT

_____

_____

_____

_____

_____

_____

_____

STRESS LEVEL

○ Fried
○ A mixed bag
○ Could vaguely imagine being calm

○ Cucumber cool
○ I own this town

This made me smile: _____

TODAY'S MENU FEATURED

BREAKFAST
_____
_____
_____

LUNCH
_____
_____
_____

DINNER
_____
_____
_____

SNACKS
_____
_____
_____

WATER _____ OZ

My most brilliant choice today: _____

I could use a do-over on this one: _____

I'll make tomorrow even more awesome by: _____
_____
_____

Date: _____ (S) (M) (T) (W) (Th) (F) (S)

WORKOUT

- O Cardio
- O Strength
- O Yoga
- O Other: _____

- O Pilates
- O Walk
- O Swim

- O Run
- O Bike

WORKED THESE ASSETS

- O Chest
- O Shoulders

- O Back
- O Arms

- O Legs
- O Abs

How'd it go?   😍   🙂   😐   🙁   😵

Details: _____

_____

_____

_____

_____

BONUS MOVES

- O Took the stairs
- O Added steps
- O Went for a walking meeting

- O Walked the dog
- O Went dancing with friends
- O Other: _____

MOOD & ENERGY REPORT

_____

_____

_____

_____

_____

_____

_____

STRESS LEVEL

○ Fried
○ A mixed bag
○ Could vaguely imagine being calm

○ Cucumber cool
○ I own this town

This made me smile: _____

TODAY'S MENU FEATURED

BREAKFAST
_____
_____
_____

LUNCH
_____
_____
_____

DINNER
_____
_____
_____

SNACKS
_____
_____
_____

WATER _____ OZ

My most brilliant choice today: _____
I could use a do-over on this one: _____
I'll make tomorrow even more awesome by: _____
_____
_____

Date: _____   (S) (M) (T) (W) (Th) (F) (S)

WORKOUT

- ◯ Cardio
- ◯ Strength
- ◯ Yoga
- ◯ Other: _____

- ◯ Pilates
- ◯ Walk
- ◯ Swim

- ◯ Run
- ◯ Bike

WORKED THESE ASSETS

- ◯ Chest
- ◯ Shoulders

- ◯ Back
- ◯ Arms

- ◯ Legs
- ◯ Abs

How'd it go? (☺) (☺) (☺) (☹) (☒)

Details: _____

_____

_____

_____

_____

BONUS MOVES

- ◯ Took the stairs
- ◯ Added steps
- ◯ Went for a walking meeting

- ◯ Walked the dog
- ◯ Went dancing with friends
- ◯ Other: _____

MOOD & ENERGY REPORT

_____

_____

_____

_____

_____

_____

_____

◯ Fried   ◯ Cucumber cool
◯ A mixed bag   ◯ I own this town
◯ Could vaguely imagine
  being calm

This made me smile: _____

TODAY'S MENU FEATURED

BREAKFAST
_____
_____
_____

LUNCH
_____
_____
_____

DINNER
_____
_____
_____

SNACKS
_____
_____
_____

WATER _____ OZ

My most brilliant choice today: _____

I could use a do-over on this one: _____

I'll make tomorrow even more awesome by: _____

_____
_____

Date: _____   (S) (M) (T) (W) (Th) (F) (S)

WORKOUT

- ◯ Cardio
- ◯ Strength
- ◯ Yoga
- ◯ Other: _____

- ◯ Pilates
- ◯ Walk
- ◯ Swim

- ◯ Run
- ◯ Bike

WORKED THESE ASSETS

- ◯ Chest
- ◯ Shoulders

- ◯ Back
- ◯ Arms

- ◯ Legs
- ◯ Abs

How'd it go?   (😍)   (🙂)   (😐)   (🙁)   (😵)

Details: _____

_____

_____

_____

_____

BONUS MOVES

- ◯ Took the stairs
- ◯ Added steps
- ◯ Went for a walking meeting

- ◯ Walked the dog
- ◯ Went dancing with friends
- ◯ Other: _____

MOOD & ENERGY REPORT

_____

_____

_____

_____

_____

_____

_____

○ Fried
○ A mixed bag
○ Could vaguely imagine being calm

○ Cucumber cool
○ I own this town

This made me smile: _____

TODAY'S MENU FEATURED

BREAKFAST
_____
_____
_____

LUNCH
_____
_____
_____

DINNER
_____
_____
_____

SNACKS
_____
_____
_____

WATER _____ OZ

My most brilliant choice today: _____

I could use a do-over on this one: _____

I'll make tomorrow even more awesome by: _____

_____

_____

Date: _____ (S) (M) (T) (W) (Th) (F) (S)

WORKOUT

- ◯ Cardio
- ◯ Strength
- ◯ Yoga
- ◯ Other: _____

- ◯ Pilates
- ◯ Walk
- ◯ Swim

- ◯ Run
- ◯ Bike

WORKED THESE ASSETS

- ◯ Chest
- ◯ Shoulders

- ◯ Back
- ◯ Arms

- ◯ Legs
- ◯ Abs

How'd it go?   (☺)   (☺)   (😐)   (🙁)   (😵)

Details: _____

_____

_____

_____

_____

BONUS MOVES

- ◯ Took the stairs
- ◯ Added steps
- ◯ Went for a walking meeting

- ◯ Walked the dog
- ◯ Went dancing with friends
- ◯ Other: _____

MOOD & ENERGY REPORT

_____

_____

_____

_____

_____

_____

_____

STRESS LEVEL

- ◯ Fried
- ◯ A mixed bag
- ◯ Could vaguely imagine being calm

- ◯ Cucumber cool
- ◯ I own this town

This made me smile: _____

TODAY'S MENU FEATURED

BREAKFAST
_____
_____
_____

LUNCH
_____
_____
_____

DINNER
_____
_____
_____

SNACKS
_____
_____
_____

WATER _____ OZ

My most brilliant choice today: _____

I could use a do-over on this one: _____

I'll make tomorrow even more awesome by: _____
_____
_____

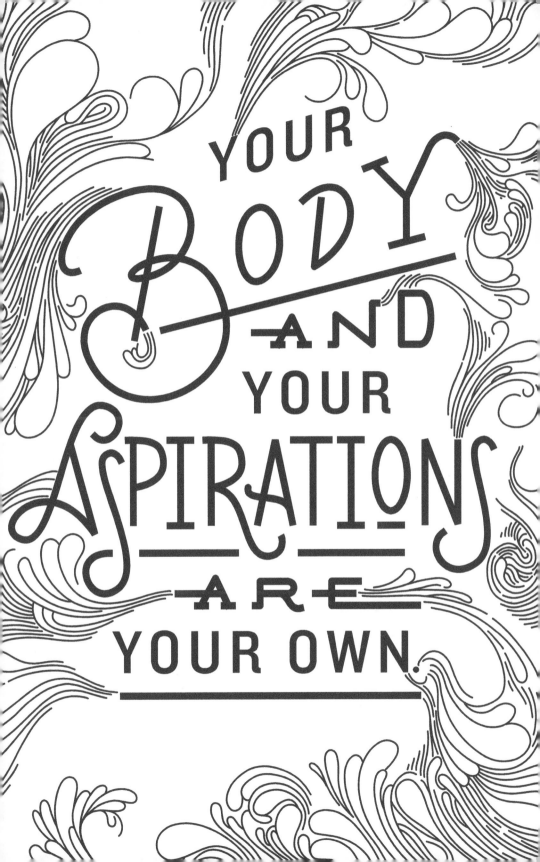

Date: _____   (S) (M) (T) (W) (Th) (F) (S)

WORKOUT

- ◯ Cardio
- ◯ Strength
- ◯ Yoga
- ◯ Other: _____

- ◯ Pilates
- ◯ Walk
- ◯ Swim

- ◯ Run
- ◯ Bike

WORKED THESE ASSETS

- ◯ Chest
- ◯ Shoulders

- ◯ Back
- ◯ Arms

- ◯ Legs
- ◯ Abs

How'd it go?   😍   🙂   😐   🙁   😵

Details: _____

_____

_____

_____

_____

BONUS MOVES

- ◯ Took the stairs
- ◯ Added steps
- ◯ Went for a walking meeting

- ◯ Walked the dog
- ◯ Went dancing with friends
- ◯ Other: _____

MOOD & ENERGY REPORT

_____

_____

_____

_____

_____

_____

_____

○ Fried
○ A mixed bag
○ Could vaguely imagine being calm

○ Cucumber cool
○ I own this town

This made me smile: _____

TODAY'S MENU FEATURED

BREAKFAST
_____
_____
_____

LUNCH
_____
_____
_____

DINNER
_____
_____
_____

SNACKS
_____
_____
_____

WATER _____ OZ

My most brilliant choice today: _____

I could use a do-over on this one: _____

I'll make tomorrow even more awesome by: _____

_____

_____

Date: _____ (S) (M) (T) (W) (Th) (F) (S)

WORKOUT

- ◯ Cardio
- ◯ Strength
- ◯ Yoga
- ◯ Other: _____

- ◯ Pilates
- ◯ Walk
- ◯ Swim

- ◯ Run
- ◯ Bike

WORKED THESE ASSETS

- ◯ Chest
- ◯ Shoulders

- ◯ Back
- ◯ Arms

- ◯ Legs
- ◯ Abs

How'd it go?   (♥‿♥)   (^‿^)   (˘_˘)   (¬_¬)   (x_x)

Details: _____

_____

_____

_____

_____

BONUS MOVES

- ◯ Took the stairs
- ◯ Added steps
- ◯ Went for a walking meeting

- ◯ Walked the dog
- ◯ Went dancing with friends
- ◯ Other: _____

MOOD & ENERGY REPORT

_____

_____

_____

_____

_____

_____

_____

STRESS LEVEL

- ○ Fried
- ○ A mixed bag
- ○ Could vaguely imagine being calm

- ○ Cucumber cool
- ○ I own this town

This made me smile: _____

TODAY'S MENU FEATURED

BREAKFAST
_____
_____
_____

LUNCH
_____
_____
_____

DINNER
_____
_____
_____

SNACKS
_____
_____
_____

WATER _____ OZ

My most brilliant choice today: _____

I could use a do-over on this one: _____

I'll make tomorrow even more awesome by: _____

_____

_____

Date: _____ (S) (M) (T) (W) (Th) (F) (S)

WORKOUT

- ◯ Cardio
- ◯ Strength
- ◯ Yoga
- ◯ Other: _____

- ◯ Pilates
- ◯ Walk
- ◯ Swim

- ◯ Run
- ◯ Bike

WORKED THESE ASSETS

- ◯ Chest
- ◯ Shoulders

- ◯ Back
- ◯ Arms

- ◯ Legs
- ◯ Abs

How'd it go?   😍   🙂   😐   🙁   😵

Details: _____

_____

_____

_____

_____

BONUS MOVES

- ◯ Took the stairs
- ◯ Added steps
- ◯ Went for a walking meeting

- ◯ Walked the dog
- ◯ Went dancing with friends
- ◯ Other: _____

MOOD & ENERGY REPORT

_____

_____

_____

_____

_____

_____

_____

STRESS LEVEL

- ◯ Fried
- ◯ A mixed bag
- ◯ Could vaguely imagine being calm

- ◯ Cucumber cool
- ◯ I own this town

This made me smile: _____

TODAY'S MENU FEATURED

BREAKFAST
_____
_____
_____

LUNCH
_____
_____
_____

DINNER
_____
_____
_____

SNACKS
_____
_____
_____

WATER _____ OZ

My most brilliant choice today: _____

I could use a do-over on this one: _____

I'll make tomorrow even more awesome by: _____

_____

_____

Date: _____   (S) (M) (T) (W) (Th) (F) (S)

WORKOUT

- ◯ Cardio
- ◯ Strength
- ◯ Yoga
- ◯ Other: _____

- ◯ Pilates
- ◯ Walk
- ◯ Swim

- ◯ Run
- ◯ Bike

WORKED THESE ASSETS

- ◯ Chest
- ◯ Shoulders

- ◯ Back
- ◯ Arms

- ◯ Legs
- ◯ Abs

How'd it go?   😍   🙂   😐   🙁   😵

Details: _____
_____
_____
_____
_____

BONUS MOVES

- ◯ Took the stairs
- ◯ Added steps
- ◯ Went for a walking meeting

- ◯ Walked the dog
- ◯ Went dancing with friends
- ◯ Other: _____

MOOD & ENERGY REPORT

_____
_____
_____
_____
_____
_____
_____

STRESS LEVEL

○ Fried
○ A mixed bag
○ Could vaguely imagine being calm

○ Cucumber cool
○ I own this town

This made me smile: _____

TODAY'S MENU FEATURED

BREAKFAST
_____
_____
_____

LUNCH
_____
_____
_____

DINNER
_____
_____
_____

SNACKS
_____
_____
_____

WATER _____ OZ

My most brilliant choice today: _____

I could use a do-over on this one: _____

I'll make tomorrow even more awesome by: _____

_____

_____

Date: _____ Ⓢ Ⓜ Ⓣ Ⓦ Ⓣⓗ Ⓕ Ⓢ

WORKOUT

- ◯ Cardio
- ◯ Strength
- ◯ Yoga
- ◯ Other: _____

- ◯ Pilates
- ◯ Walk
- ◯ Swim

- ◯ Run
- ◯ Bike

WORKED THESE ASSETS

- ◯ Chest
- ◯ Shoulders

- ◯ Back
- ◯ Arms

- ◯ Legs
- ◯ Abs

How'd it go? 😍 🙂 😐 🙁 😵

Details: _____

_____

_____

_____

_____

BONUS MOVES

- ◯ Took the stairs
- ◯ Added steps
- ◯ Went for a walking meeting

- ◯ Walked the dog
- ◯ Went dancing with friends
- ◯ Other: _____

MOOD & ENERGY REPORT

_____

_____

_____

_____

_____

_____

_____

○ Fried
○ A mixed bag
○ Could vaguely imagine being calm

○ Cucumber cool
○ I own this town

This made me smile: _____

TODAY'S MENU FEATURED

BREAKFAST
_____
_____
_____

LUNCH
_____
_____
_____

DINNER
_____
_____
_____

SNACKS
_____
_____
_____

WATER _____ OZ

My most brilliant choice today: _____

I could use a do-over on this one: _____

I'll make tomorrow even more awesome by: _____

_____

_____

Date: _____   (S) (M) (T) (W) (Th) (F) (S)

WORKOUT

- ◯ Cardio
- ◯ Strength
- ◯ Yoga
- ◯ Other: _____

- ◯ Pilates
- ◯ Walk
- ◯ Swim

- ◯ Run
- ◯ Bike

WORKED THESE ASSETS

- ◯ Chest
- ◯ Shoulders

- ◯ Back
- ◯ Arms

- ◯ Legs
- ◯ Abs

How'd it go?   😍   🙂   😐   🙁   😵

Details: _____
_____
_____
_____
_____

BONUS MOVES

- ◯ Took the stairs
- ◯ Added steps
- ◯ Went for a walking meeting

- ◯ Walked the dog
- ◯ Went dancing with friends
- ◯ Other: _____

MOOD & ENERGY REPORT

_____
_____
_____
_____
_____
_____
_____

STRESS LEVEL

○ Fried
○ A mixed bag
○ Could vaguely imagine
   being calm

○ Cucumber cool
○ I own this town

This made me smile: _____

TODAY'S MENU FEATURED

BREAKFAST
_____
_____
_____

LUNCH
_____
_____
_____

DINNER
_____
_____
_____

SNACKS
_____
_____
_____

WATER _____ OZ

My most brilliant choice today: _____

I could use a do-over on this one: _____

I'll make tomorrow even more awesome by: _____

_____

_____

Date: _____   (S) (M) (T) (W) (Th) (F) (S)

WORKOUT

○ Cardio   ○ Pilates   ○ Run
○ Strength   ○ Walk   ○ Bike
○ Yoga   ○ Swim
○ Other: _____

WORKED THESE ASSETS

○ Chest   ○ Back   ○ Legs
○ Shoulders   ○ Arms   ○ Abs

How'd it go?   😍   🙂   😐   🙁   😵

Details: _____
_____
_____
_____
_____

BONUS MOVES

○ Took the stairs   ○ Walked the dog
○ Added steps   ○ Went dancing with friends
○ Went for a walking meeting   ○ Other: _____

MOOD & ENERGY REPORT

_____
_____
_____
_____
_____
_____
_____

○ Fried
○ A mixed bag
○ Could vaguely imagine being calm

○ Cucumber cool
○ I own this town

This made me smile: _____

TODAY'S MENU FEATURED

BREAKFAST
_____
_____
_____

LUNCH
_____
_____
_____

DINNER
_____
_____
_____

SNACKS
_____
_____
_____

WATER _____ OZ

My most brilliant choice today: _____

I could use a do-over on this one: _____

I'll make tomorrow even more awesome by: _____

_____

_____

Date: _____ (S) (M) (T) (W) (Th) (F) (S)

WORKOUT

- ◯ Cardio
- ◯ Strength
- ◯ Yoga
- ◯ Other: _____

- ◯ Pilates
- ◯ Walk
- ◯ Swim

- ◯ Run
- ◯ Bike

WORKED THESE ASSETS

- ◯ Chest
- ◯ Shoulders

- ◯ Back
- ◯ Arms

- ◯ Legs
- ◯ Abs

How'd it go?   😍   🙂   😐   🙁   😵

Details: _____
_____
_____
_____
_____

BONUS MOVES

- ◯ Took the stairs
- ◯ Added steps
- ◯ Went for a walking meeting

- ◯ Walked the dog
- ◯ Went dancing with friends
- ◯ Other: _____

MOOD & ENERGY REPORT

_____
_____
_____
_____
_____
_____

STRESS LEVEL

○ Fried
○ A mixed bag
○ Could vaguely imagine being calm

○ Cucumber cool
○ I own this town

This made me smile: _____

TODAY'S MENU FEATURED

BREAKFAST
_____
_____
_____

LUNCH
_____
_____
_____

DINNER
_____
_____
_____

SNACKS
_____
_____
_____

WATER _____ OZ

My most brilliant choice today: _____

I could use a do-over on this one: _____

I'll make tomorrow even more awesome by: _____

_____

_____

Date: _____   (S) (M) (T) (W) (Th) (F) (S)

WORKOUT

- ◯ Cardio
- ◯ Strength
- ◯ Yoga
- ◯ Other: _____

- ◯ Pilates
- ◯ Walk
- ◯ Swim

- ◯ Run
- ◯ Bike

WORKED THESE ASSETS

- ◯ Chest
- ◯ Shoulders

- ◯ Back
- ◯ Arms

- ◯ Legs
- ◯ Abs

How'd it go?   😍 🙂 😐 🙁 😵

Details: _____

_____

_____

_____

_____

BONUS MOVES

- ◯ Took the stairs
- ◯ Added steps
- ◯ Went for a walking meeting

- ◯ Walked the dog
- ◯ Went dancing with friends
- ◯ Other: _____

MOOD & ENERGY REPORT

_____

_____

_____

_____

_____

_____

_____

STRESS LEVEL

○ Fried
○ A mixed bag
○ Could vaguely imagine being calm

○ Cucumber cool
○ I own this town

This made me smile: _____

TODAY'S MENU FEATURED

BREAKFAST
_____
_____
_____

LUNCH
_____
_____
_____

DINNER
_____
_____
_____

SNACKS
_____
_____
_____

WATER _____ OZ

My most brilliant choice today: _____
I could use a do-over on this one: _____
I'll make tomorrow even more awesome by: _____
_____
_____

Date: _____   (S) (M) (T) (W) (Th) (F) (S)

WORKOUT

○ Cardio   ○ Pilates   ○ Run
○ Strength   ○ Walk   ○ Bike
○ Yoga   ○ Swim
○ Other: _____

WORKED THESE ASSETS

○ Chest   ○ Back   ○ Legs
○ Shoulders   ○ Arms   ○ Abs

How'd it go?   😍   🙂   😐   🙁   😵

Details: _____
_____
_____
_____
_____

BONUS MOVES

○ Took the stairs   ○ Walked the dog
○ Added steps   ○ Went dancing with friends
○ Went for a walking meeting   ○ Other: _____

MOOD & ENERGY REPORT

_____
_____
_____
_____
_____
_____
_____

◯ Fried   ◯ Cucumber cool
◯ A mixed bag   ◯ I own this town
◯ Could vaguely imagine
   being calm

This made me smile: _____

TODAY'S MENU FEATURED

BREAKFAST
_____
_____
_____

LUNCH
_____
_____
_____

DINNER
_____
_____
_____

SNACKS
_____
_____
_____

WATER _____ OZ

My most brilliant choice today: _____
I could use a do-over on this one: _____
I'll make tomorrow even more awesome by: _____
_____
_____

Date: _____ S M T W Th F S

WORKOUT

- ◯ Cardio
- ◯ Strength
- ◯ Yoga
- ◯ Other: _____

- ◯ Pilates
- ◯ Walk
- ◯ Swim

- ◯ Run
- ◯ Bike

WORKED THESE ASSETS

- ◯ Chest
- ◯ Shoulders

- ◯ Back
- ◯ Arms

- ◯ Legs
- ◯ Abs

How'd it go? 😍 🙂 😐 🙁 😵

Details: _____

_____

_____

_____

_____

BONUS MOVES

- ◯ Took the stairs
- ◯ Added steps
- ◯ Went for a walking meeting

- ◯ Walked the dog
- ◯ Went dancing with friends
- ◯ Other: _____

MOOD & ENERGY REPORT

_____

_____

_____

_____

_____

_____

_____

STRESS LEVEL

○ Fried
○ A mixed bag
○ Could vaguely imagine being calm

○ Cucumber cool
○ I own this town

This made me smile: _____

TODAY'S MENU FEATURED

BREAKFAST
_____
_____
_____

LUNCH
_____
_____
_____

DINNER
_____
_____
_____

SNACKS
_____
_____
_____

WATER _____ OZ

My most brilliant choice today: _____

I could use a do-over on this one: _____

I'll make tomorrow even more awesome by: _____

_____

_____

Date: _____ (S) (M) (T) (W) (Th) (F) (S)

WORKOUT

- ◯ Cardio   ◯ Pilates   ◯ Run
- ◯ Strength   ◯ Walk   ◯ Bike
- ◯ Yoga   ◯ Swim
- ◯ Other: _____

WORKED THESE ASSETS

- ◯ Chest   ◯ Back   ◯ Legs
- ◯ Shoulders   ◯ Arms   ◯ Abs

How'd it go?   😍   🙂   😐   🙁   😵

Details: _____

_____

_____

_____

_____

BONUS MOVES

- ◯ Took the stairs   ◯ Walked the dog
- ◯ Added steps   ◯ Went dancing with friends
- ◯ Went for a walking meeting   ◯ Other: _____

MOOD & ENERGY REPORT

_____

_____

_____

_____

_____

_____

_____

STRESS LEVEL

○ Fried
○ A mixed bag
○ Could vaguely imagine being calm

○ Cucumber cool
○ I own this town

This made me smile: _____

TODAY'S MENU FEATURED

BREAKFAST
_____
_____
_____

LUNCH
_____
_____
_____

DINNER
_____
_____
_____

SNACKS
_____
_____
_____

WATER _____ OZ

My most brilliant choice today: _____
I could use a do-over on this one: _____
I'll make tomorrow even more awesome by: _____
_____
_____

Date: _____ (S) (M) (T) (W) (Th) (F) (S)

WORKOUT

- ◯ Cardio
- ◯ Strength
- ◯ Yoga
- ◯ Other: _____

- ◯ Pilates
- ◯ Walk
- ◯ Swim

- ◯ Run
- ◯ Bike

WORKED THESE ASSETS

- ◯ Chest
- ◯ Shoulders

- ◯ Back
- ◯ Arms

- ◯ Legs
- ◯ Abs

How'd it go?   😍   🙂   😐   🙁   😵

Details: _____

_____

_____

_____

_____

BONUS MOVES

- ◯ Took the stairs
- ◯ Added steps
- ◯ Went for a walking meeting

- ◯ Walked the dog
- ◯ Went dancing with friends
- ◯ Other: _____

MOOD & ENERGY REPORT

_____

_____

_____

_____

_____

_____

_____

○ Fried
○ A mixed bag
○ Could vaguely imagine being calm

○ Cucumber cool
○ I own this town

This made me smile: _____

TODAY'S MENU FEATURED

BREAKFAST
_____
_____
_____

LUNCH
_____
_____
_____

DINNER
_____
_____
_____

SNACKS
_____
_____
_____

WATER _____ OZ

My most brilliant choice today: _____

I could use a do-over on this one: _____

I'll make tomorrow even more awesome by: _____

_____

_____

Date: _____ S M T W Th F S

WORKOUT

○ Cardio   ○ Pilates   ○ Run
○ Strength ○ Walk   ○ Bike
○ Yoga   ○ Swim
○ Other: _____

WORKED THESE ASSETS

○ Chest   ○ Back   ○ Legs
○ Shoulders ○ Arms   ○ Abs

How'd it go?   😍   🙂   😐   🙁   😵

Details: _____
_____
_____
_____
_____

BONUS MOVES

○ Took the stairs   ○ Walked the dog
○ Added steps   ○ Went dancing with friends
○ Went for a walking meeting ○ Other: _____

MOOD & ENERGY REPORT

_____
_____
_____
_____
_____
_____
_____

STRESS LEVEL

◯ Fried
◯ A mixed bag
◯ Could vaguely imagine being calm

◯ Cucumber cool
◯ I own this town

This made me smile: _____

TODAY'S MENU FEATURED

BREAKFAST
_____
_____
_____

LUNCH
_____
_____
_____

DINNER
_____
_____
_____

SNACKS
_____
_____
_____

WATER _____ OZ

My most brilliant choice today: _____

I could use a do-over on this one: _____

I'll make tomorrow even more awesome by: _____

_____

_____

Date: _____ (S) (M) (T) (W) (Th) (F) (S)

WORKOUT

- ◯ Cardio
- ◯ Strength
- ◯ Yoga
- ◯ Other: _____

- ◯ Pilates
- ◯ Walk
- ◯ Swim

- ◯ Run
- ◯ Bike

WORKED THESE ASSETS

- ◯ Chest
- ◯ Shoulders

- ◯ Back
- ◯ Arms

- ◯ Legs
- ◯ Abs

How'd it go?   😍   🙂   😐   🙁   😵

Details: _____

_____

_____

_____

_____

BONUS MOVES

- ◯ Took the stairs
- ◯ Added steps
- ◯ Went for a walking meeting

- ◯ Walked the dog
- ◯ Went dancing with friends
- ◯ Other: _____

MOOD & ENERGY REPORT

_____

_____

_____

_____

_____

_____

_____

○ Fried
○ A mixed bag
○ Could vaguely imagine being calm

○ Cucumber cool
○ I own this town

This made me smile: _____

TODAY'S MENU FEATURED

BREAKFAST
_____
_____
_____

LUNCH
_____
_____
_____

DINNER
_____
_____
_____

SNACKS
_____
_____
_____

WATER _____ OZ

My most brilliant choice today: _____

I could use a do-over on this one: _____

I'll make tomorrow even more awesome by: _____

_____
_____

PROGRESS ISN'T LINEAR.

YOUR PATH WILL HAVE

BUT UPS AND DOWNS,

YOU

GET TO DECIDE

AT WHAT SPEED YOU RACE

TOWARD

YOUR GOALS.

Date: _____   (S) (M) (T) (W) (Th) (F) (S)

WORKOUT

- ◯ Cardio
- ◯ Strength
- ◯ Yoga
- ◯ Other: _____

- ◯ Pilates
- ◯ Walk
- ◯ Swim

- ◯ Run
- ◯ Bike

WORKED THESE ASSETS

- ◯ Chest
- ◯ Shoulders

- ◯ Back
- ◯ Arms

- ◯ Legs
- ◯ Abs

How'd it go?   😍   🙂   😐   🙁   😵

Details: _____

_____

_____

_____

_____

BONUS MOVES

- ◯ Took the stairs
- ◯ Added steps
- ◯ Went for a walking meeting

- ◯ Walked the dog
- ◯ Went dancing with friends
- ◯ Other: _____

MOOD & ENERGY REPORT

_____

_____

_____

_____

_____

_____

_____

STRESS LEVEL

○ Fried
○ A mixed bag
○ Could vaguely imagine being calm

○ Cucumber cool
○ I own this town

This made me smile: _____

TODAY'S MENU FEATURED

BREAKFAST
_____
_____
_____

LUNCH
_____
_____
_____

DINNER
_____
_____
_____

SNACKS
_____
_____
_____

WATER _____ OZ

My most brilliant choice today: _____

I could use a do-over on this one: _____

I'll make tomorrow even more awesome by: _____

_____

_____

Date: _____   (S) (M) (T) (W) (Th) (F) (S)

WORKOUT

○ Cardio   ○ Pilates   ○ Run
○ Strength   ○ Walk   ○ Bike
○ Yoga   ○ Swim
○ Other: _____

WORKED THESE ASSETS

○ Chest   ○ Back   ○ Legs
○ Shoulders   ○ Arms   ○ Abs

How'd it go?   😍   🙂   😐   🙁   😣

Details: _____
_____
_____
_____
_____

BONUS MOVES

○ Took the stairs   ○ Walked the dog
○ Added steps   ○ Went dancing with friends
○ Went for a walking meeting ○ Other: _____

MOOD & ENERGY REPORT

_____
_____
_____
_____
_____
_____
_____

STRESS LEVEL

○ Fried
○ A mixed bag
○ Could vaguely imagine being calm

○ Cucumber cool
○ I own this town

This made me smile: _____

TODAY'S MENU FEATURED

BREAKFAST
_____
_____
_____

LUNCH
_____
_____
_____

DINNER
_____
_____
_____

SNACKS
_____
_____
_____

WATER _____ OZ

My most brilliant choice today: _____

I could use a do-over on this one: _____

I'll make tomorrow even more awesome by: _____

_____
_____

Date: _____ (S) (M) (T) (W) (Th) (F) (S)

WORKOUT

○ Cardio   ○ Pilates   ○ Run
○ Strength   ○ Walk   ○ Bike
○ Yoga   ○ Swim
○ Other: _____

WORKED THESE ASSETS

○ Chest   ○ Back   ○ Legs
○ Shoulders   ○ Arms   ○ Abs

How'd it go?   😍   🙂   😐   🙁   😵

Details: _____
_____
_____
_____
_____

BONUS MOVES

○ Took the stairs   ○ Walked the dog
○ Added steps   ○ Went dancing with friends
○ Went for a walking meeting   ○ Other: _____

MOOD & ENERGY REPORT

_____
_____
_____
_____
_____
_____
_____

○ Fried
○ A mixed bag
○ Could vaguely imagine being calm

○ Cucumber cool
○ I own this town

This made me smile: _____

TODAY'S MENU FEATURED

BREAKFAST
_____
_____
_____

LUNCH
_____
_____
_____

DINNER
_____
_____
_____

SNACKS
_____
_____
_____

WATER _____ OZ

My most brilliant choice today: _____

I could use a do-over on this one: _____

I'll make tomorrow even more awesome by: _____

_____

_____

Date: _____   (S) (M) (T) (W) (Th) (F) (S)

WORKOUT

- ◯ Cardio
- ◯ Strength
- ◯ Yoga
- ◯ Other: _____

- ◯ Pilates
- ◯ Walk
- ◯ Swim

- ◯ Run
- ◯ Bike

WORKED THESE ASSETS

- ◯ Chest
- ◯ Shoulders

- ◯ Back
- ◯ Arms

- ◯ Legs
- ◯ Abs

How'd it go?   😍   🙂   😐   🙁   😵

Details: _____
_____
_____
_____
_____

BONUS MOVES

- ◯ Took the stairs
- ◯ Added steps
- ◯ Went for a walking meeting

- ◯ Walked the dog
- ◯ Went dancing with friends
- ◯ Other: _____

MOOD & ENERGY REPORT

_____
_____
_____
_____
_____
_____
_____

◯ Fried
◯ A mixed bag
◯ Could vaguely imagine being calm

◯ Cucumber cool
◯ I own this town

This made me smile: _____

TODAY'S MENU FEATURED

BREAKFAST
_____
_____
_____

LUNCH
_____
_____
_____

DINNER
_____
_____
_____

SNACKS
_____
_____
_____

WATER _____ OZ

My most brilliant choice today: _____

I could use a do-over on this one: _____

I'll make tomorrow even more awesome by: _____

_____

_____

Date: _____   (S) (M) (T) (W) (Th) (F) (S)

WORKOUT

- ◯ Cardio
- ◯ Strength
- ◯ Yoga
- ◯ Other: _____

- ◯ Pilates
- ◯ Walk
- ◯ Swim

- ◯ Run
- ◯ Bike

WORKED THESE ASSETS

- ◯ Chest
- ◯ Shoulders

- ◯ Back
- ◯ Arms

- ◯ Legs
- ◯ Abs

How'd it go?   😍   🙂   😐   🙁   😵

Details: _____

_____

_____

_____

_____

BONUS MOVES

- ◯ Took the stairs
- ◯ Added steps
- ◯ Went for a walking meeting

- ◯ Walked the dog
- ◯ Went dancing with friends
- ◯ Other: _____

MOOD & ENERGY REPORT

_____

_____

_____

_____

_____

_____

STRESS LEVEL

○ Fried
○ A mixed bag
○ Could vaguely imagine being calm

○ Cucumber cool
○ I own this town

This made me smile: _____

TODAY'S MENU FEATURED

BREAKFAST
_____
_____
_____

LUNCH
_____
_____
_____

DINNER
_____
_____
_____

SNACKS
_____
_____
_____

WATER _____ OZ

My most brilliant choice today: _____
I could use a do-over on this one: _____
I'll make tomorrow even more awesome by: _____
_____
_____

Date: _____   (S) (M) (T) (W) (Th) (F) (S)

WORKOUT

○ Cardio   ○ Pilates   ○ Run
○ Strength   ○ Walk   ○ Bike
○ Yoga   ○ Swim
○ Other: _____

WORKED THESE ASSETS

○ Chest   ○ Back   ○ Legs
○ Shoulders   ○ Arms   ○ Abs

How'd it go?   😍   🙂   😐   🙁   😵

Details: _____
_____
_____
_____
_____

BONUS MOVES

○ Took the stairs   ○ Walked the dog
○ Added steps   ○ Went dancing with friends
○ Went for a walking meeting   ○ Other: _____

MOOD & ENERGY REPORT

_____
_____
_____
_____
_____
_____
_____

○ Fried   ○ Cucumber cool
○ A mixed bag   ○ I own this town
○ Could vaguely imagine
  being calm

This made me smile: _____

TODAY'S MENU FEATURED

BREAKFAST
_____
_____
_____

LUNCH
_____
_____
_____

DINNER
_____
_____
_____

SNACKS
_____
_____
_____

WATER _____ OZ

My most brilliant choice today: _____

I could use a do-over on this one: _____

I'll make tomorrow even more awesome by: _____

_____

_____

Date: _____ (S) (M) (T) (W) (Th) (F) (S)

WORKOUT

- ◯ Cardio
- ◯ Strength
- ◯ Yoga
- ◯ Other: _____

- ◯ Pilates
- ◯ Walk
- ◯ Swim

- ◯ Run
- ◯ Bike

WORKED THESE ASSETS

- ◯ Chest
- ◯ Shoulders

- ◯ Back
- ◯ Arms

- ◯ Legs
- ◯ Abs

How'd it go?   😍   🙂   😐   🙁   😵

Details: _____

_____

_____

_____

_____

BONUS MOVES

- ◯ Took the stairs
- ◯ Added steps
- ◯ Went for a walking meeting

- ◯ Walked the dog
- ◯ Went dancing with friends
- ◯ Other: _____

MOOD & ENERGY REPORT

_____

_____

_____

_____

_____

_____

_____

○ Fried
○ A mixed bag
○ Could vaguely imagine being calm

○ Cucumber cool
○ I own this town

This made me smile: _____

TODAY'S MENU FEATURED

BREAKFAST
_____
_____
_____

LUNCH
_____
_____
_____

DINNER
_____
_____
_____

SNACKS
_____
_____
_____

WATER _____ OZ

My most brilliant choice today: _____

I could use a do-over on this one: _____

I'll make tomorrow even more awesome by: _____

_____

_____

Date: _____   (S) (M) (T) (W) (Th) (F) (S)

WORKOUT

- ⭘ Cardio
- ⭘ Strength
- ⭘ Yoga
- ⭘ Other: _____

- ⭘ Pilates
- ⭘ Walk
- ⭘ Swim

- ⭘ Run
- ⭘ Bike

WORKED THESE ASSETS

- ⭘ Chest
- ⭘ Shoulders

- ⭘ Back
- ⭘ Arms

- ⭘ Legs
- ⭘ Abs

How'd it go?   😍   🙂   😐   🙁   😵

Details: _____

_____

_____

_____

_____

BONUS MOVES

- ⭘ Took the stairs
- ⭘ Added steps
- ⭘ Went for a walking meeting

- ⭘ Walked the dog
- ⭘ Went dancing with friends
- ⭘ Other: _____

MOOD & ENERGY REPORT

_____

_____

_____

_____

_____

_____

_____

STRESS LEVEL

- ◯ Fried
- ◯ A mixed bag
- ◯ Could vaguely imagine being calm

- ◯ Cucumber cool
- ◯ I own this town

This made me smile: _____

TODAY'S MENU FEATURED

BREAKFAST
_____
_____
_____

LUNCH
_____
_____
_____

DINNER
_____
_____
_____

SNACKS
_____
_____
_____

WATER _____ OZ

My most brilliant choice today: _____

I could use a do-over on this one: _____

I'll make tomorrow even more awesome by: _____

_____

_____

Date: _____   (S) (M) (T) (W) (Th) (F) (S)

WORKOUT

○ Cardio   ○ Pilates   ○ Run
○ Strength   ○ Walk   ○ Bike
○ Yoga   ○ Swim
○ Other: _____

WORKED THESE ASSETS

○ Chest   ○ Back   ○ Legs
○ Shoulders   ○ Arms   ○ Abs

How'd it go?   😍   🙂   😐   🙁   😵

Details: _____
_____
_____
_____
_____

BONUS MOVES

○ Took the stairs   ○ Walked the dog
○ Added steps   ○ Went dancing with friends
○ Went for a walking meeting ○ Other: _____

MOOD & ENERGY REPORT

_____
_____
_____
_____
_____
_____
_____

STRESS LEVEL

◯ Fried
◯ A mixed bag
◯ Could vaguely imagine being calm

◯ Cucumber cool
◯ I own this town

This made me smile: _____

TODAY'S MENU FEATURED

BREAKFAST
_____
_____
_____

LUNCH
_____
_____
_____

DINNER
_____
_____
_____

SNACKS
_____
_____
_____

WATER _____ OZ

My most brilliant choice today: _____

I could use a do-over on this one: _____

I'll make tomorrow even more awesome by: _____

_____

_____

Date: _____   (S) (M) (T) (W) (Th) (F) (S)

WORKOUT

- ◯ Cardio   ◯ Pilates   ◯ Run
- ◯ Strength   ◯ Walk   ◯ Bike
- ◯ Yoga   ◯ Swim
- ◯ Other: _____

WORKED THESE ASSETS

- ◯ Chest   ◯ Back   ◯ Legs
- ◯ Shoulders   ◯ Arms   ◯ Abs

How'd it go?   😍   🙂   😐   🙁   😵

Details: _____

_____

_____

_____

_____

BONUS MOVES

- ◯ Took the stairs   ◯ Walked the dog
- ◯ Added steps   ◯ Went dancing with friends
- ◯ Went for a walking meeting ◯ Other: _____

MOOD & ENERGY REPORT

_____

_____

_____

_____

_____

_____

_____

○ Fried
○ A mixed bag
○ Could vaguely imagine being calm

○ Cucumber cool
○ I own this town

This made me smile: _____

TODAY'S MENU FEATURED

BREAKFAST
_____
_____
_____

LUNCH
_____
_____
_____

DINNER
_____
_____
_____

SNACKS
_____
_____
_____

WATER _____ OZ

My most brilliant choice today: _____

I could use a do-over on this one: _____

I'll make tomorrow even more awesome by: _____

_____

_____

Date: _____   (S) (M) (T) (W) (Th) (F) (S)

WORKOUT

- ◯ Cardio
- ◯ Strength
- ◯ Yoga
- ◯ Other: _____

- ◯ Pilates
- ◯ Walk
- ◯ Swim

- ◯ Run
- ◯ Bike

WORKED THESE ASSETS

- ◯ Chest
- ◯ Shoulders

- ◯ Back
- ◯ Arms

- ◯ Legs
- ◯ Abs

How'd it go?   😍   🙂   😐   🙁   😣

Details: _____
_____
_____
_____
_____

BONUS MOVES

- ◯ Took the stairs
- ◯ Added steps
- ◯ Went for a walking meeting

- ◯ Walked the dog
- ◯ Went dancing with friends
- ◯ Other: _____

MOOD & ENERGY REPORT

_____
_____
_____
_____
_____
_____
_____

STRESS LEVEL

◯ Fried
◯ A mixed bag
◯ Could vaguely imagine
   being calm

◯ Cucumber cool
◯ I own this town

This made me smile: _____

TODAY'S MENU FEATURED

BREAKFAST
_____
_____
_____

LUNCH
_____
_____
_____

DINNER
_____
_____
_____

SNACKS
_____
_____
_____

WATER _____ OZ

My most brilliant choice today: _____

I could use a do-over on this one: _____

I'll make tomorrow even more awesome by: _____

_____

_____

Date: _____ (S) (M) (T) (W) (Th) (F) (S)

WORKOUT

- ◯ Cardio
- ◯ Strength
- ◯ Yoga
- ◯ Other: _____

- ◯ Pilates
- ◯ Walk
- ◯ Swim

- ◯ Run
- ◯ Bike

WORKED THESE ASSETS

- ◯ Chest
- ◯ Shoulders

- ◯ Back
- ◯ Arms

- ◯ Legs
- ◯ Abs

How'd it go?   😍   🙂   😐   🙁   😫

Details: _____
_____
_____
_____
_____

BONUS MOVES

- ◯ Took the stairs
- ◯ Added steps
- ◯ Went for a walking meeting

- ◯ Walked the dog
- ◯ Went dancing with friends
- ◯ Other: _____

MOOD & ENERGY REPORT

_____
_____
_____
_____
_____
_____
_____

STRESS LEVEL

○ Fried
○ A mixed bag
○ Could vaguely imagine
   being calm

○ Cucumber cool
○ I own this town

This made me smile: _____

TODAY'S MENU FEATURED

BREAKFAST
_____
_____
_____

LUNCH
_____
_____
_____

DINNER
_____
_____
_____

SNACKS
_____
_____
_____

WATER _____ OZ

My most brilliant choice today: _____

I could use a do-over on this one: _____

I'll make tomorrow even more awesome by: _____

_____

_____

Date: _____ (S) (M) (T) (W) (Th) (F) (S)

WORKOUT

- ◯ Cardio
- ◯ Strength
- ◯ Yoga
- ◯ Other: _____

- ◯ Pilates
- ◯ Walk
- ◯ Swim

- ◯ Run
- ◯ Bike

WORKED THESE ASSETS

- ◯ Chest
- ◯ Shoulders

- ◯ Back
- ◯ Arms

- ◯ Legs
- ◯ Abs

How'd it go?   😍   🙂   😐   🙁   😵

Details: _____

_____

_____

_____

_____

BONUS MOVES

- ◯ Took the stairs
- ◯ Added steps
- ◯ Went for a walking meeting

- ◯ Walked the dog
- ◯ Went dancing with friends
- ◯ Other: _____

MOOD & ENERGY REPORT

_____

_____

_____

_____

_____

_____

_____

STRESS LEVEL

○ Fried
○ A mixed bag
○ Could vaguely imagine being calm

○ Cucumber cool
○ I own this town

This made me smile: _____

TODAY'S MENU FEATURED

BREAKFAST
_____
_____
_____

LUNCH
_____
_____
_____

DINNER
_____
_____
_____

SNACKS
_____
_____
_____

WATER _____ OZ

My most brilliant choice today: _____

I could use a do-over on this one: _____

I'll make tomorrow even more awesome by: _____
_____
_____

Date: _____ ⓈⓂⓉⓌ(Th)(F)Ⓢ

WORKOUT

- ◯ Cardio
- ◯ Strength
- ◯ Yoga
- ◯ Other: _____

- ◯ Pilates
- ◯ Walk
- ◯ Swim

- ◯ Run
- ◯ Bike

WORKED THESE ASSETS

- ◯ Chest
- ◯ Shoulders

- ◯ Back
- ◯ Arms

- ◯ Legs
- ◯ Abs

How'd it go?   😍 🙂 😐 🙁 😵

Details: _____

_____

_____

_____

_____

BONUS MOVES

- ◯ Took the stairs
- ◯ Added steps
- ◯ Went for a walking meeting

- ◯ Walked the dog
- ◯ Went dancing with friends
- ◯ Other: _____

MOOD & ENERGY REPORT

_____

_____

_____

_____

_____

_____

_____

STRESS LEVEL

○ Fried
○ A mixed bag
○ Could vaguely imagine
  being calm

○ Cucumber cool
○ I own this town

This made me smile: _____

TODAY'S MENU FEATURED

BREAKFAST
_____
_____
_____

LUNCH
_____
_____
_____

DINNER
_____
_____
_____

SNACKS
_____
_____
_____

WATER _____ OZ

My most brilliant choice today: _____

I could use a do-over on this one: _____

I'll make tomorrow even more awesome by: _____

_____

_____

Date: _____   (S) (M) (T) (W) (Th) (F) (S)

WORKOUT

- ◯ Cardio
- ◯ Strength
- ◯ Yoga
- ◯ Other: _____

- ◯ Pilates
- ◯ Walk
- ◯ Swim

- ◯ Run
- ◯ Bike

WORKED THESE ASSETS

- ◯ Chest
- ◯ Shoulders

- ◯ Back
- ◯ Arms

- ◯ Legs
- ◯ Abs

How'd it go?   😍   🙂   😐   🙁   😣

Details: _____

_____

_____

_____

_____

BONUS MOVES

- ◯ Took the stairs
- ◯ Added steps
- ◯ Went for a walking meeting

- ◯ Walked the dog
- ◯ Went dancing with friends
- ◯ Other: _____

MOOD & ENERGY REPORT

_____

_____

_____

_____

_____

_____

_____

STRESS LEVEL

○ Fried
○ A mixed bag
○ Could vaguely imagine
  being calm

○ Cucumber cool
○ I own this town

This made me smile: _____

TODAY'S MENU FEATURED

BREAKFAST
_____
_____
_____

LUNCH
_____
_____
_____

DINNER
_____
_____
_____

SNACKS
_____
_____
_____

WATER _____ OZ

My most brilliant choice today: _____

I could use a do-over on this one: _____

I'll make tomorrow even more awesome by: _____

_____
_____

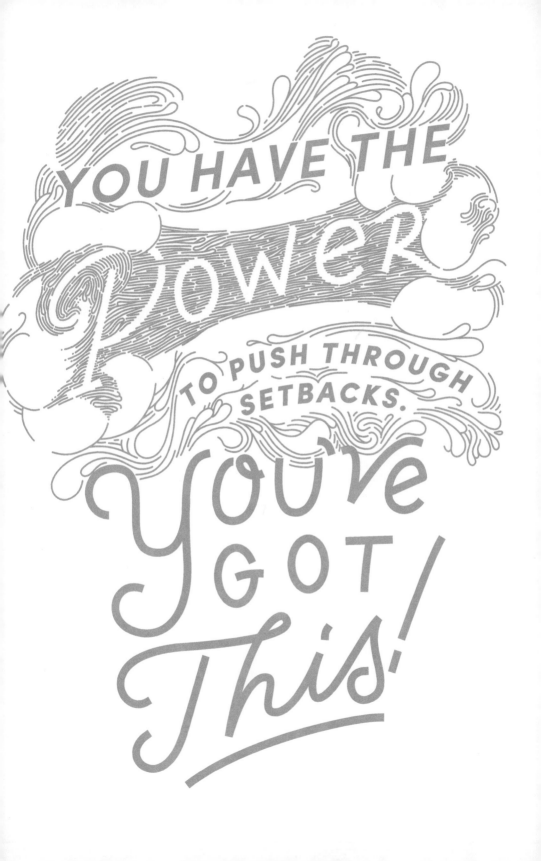

Date: _____   (S) (M) (T) (W) (Th) (F) (S)

WORKOUT

- ◯ Cardio
- ◯ Strength
- ◯ Yoga
- ◯ Other: _____

- ◯ Pilates
- ◯ Walk
- ◯ Swim

- ◯ Run
- ◯ Bike

WORKED THESE ASSETS

- ◯ Chest
- ◯ Shoulders

- ◯ Back
- ◯ Arms

- ◯ Legs
- ◯ Abs

How'd it go?   😍   🙂   😐   🙁   😵

Details: _____
_____
_____
_____
_____

BONUS MOVES

- ◯ Took the stairs
- ◯ Added steps
- ◯ Went for a walking meeting

- ◯ Walked the dog
- ◯ Went dancing with friends
- ◯ Other: _____

MOOD & ENERGY REPORT

_____
_____
_____
_____
_____
_____
_____

○ Fried

○ A mixed bag

○ Could vaguely imagine
being calm

○ Cucumber cool

○ I own this town

This made me smile: _____

TODAY'S MENU FEATURED

BREAKFAST
_____
_____
_____

LUNCH
_____
_____
_____

DINNER
_____
_____
_____

SNACKS
_____
_____
_____

WATER _____ OZ

My most brilliant choice today: _____

I could use a do-over on this one: _____

I'll make tomorrow even more awesome by: _____

_____

_____

Date: _____ (S) (M) (T) (W) (Th) (F) (S)

WORKOUT

- ○ Cardio
- ○ Strength
- ○ Yoga
- ○ Other: _____

- ○ Pilates
- ○ Walk
- ○ Swim

- ○ Run
- ○ Bike

WORKED THESE ASSETS

- ○ Chest
- ○ Shoulders

- ○ Back
- ○ Arms

- ○ Legs
- ○ Abs

How'd it go?   😍   🙂   😐   🙁   😵

Details: _____
_____
_____
_____
_____

BONUS MOVES

- ○ Took the stairs
- ○ Added steps
- ○ Went for a walking meeting

- ○ Walked the dog
- ○ Went dancing with friends
- ○ Other: _____

MOOD & ENERGY REPORT

_____
_____
_____
_____
_____
_____
_____

STRESS LEVEL

○ Fried
○ A mixed bag
○ Could vaguely imagine being calm

○ Cucumber cool
○ I own this town

This made me smile: _____

TODAY'S MENU FEATURED

BREAKFAST
_____
_____
_____

LUNCH
_____
_____
_____

DINNER
_____
_____
_____

SNACKS
_____
_____
_____

WATER _____ OZ

My most brilliant choice today: _____

I could use a do-over on this one: _____

I'll make tomorrow even more awesome by: _____

_____

_____

Date: _____   (S) (M) (T) (W) (Th) (F) (S)

WORKOUT

- ◯ Cardio
- ◯ Strength
- ◯ Yoga
- ◯ Other: _____

- ◯ Pilates
- ◯ Walk
- ◯ Swim

- ◯ Run
- ◯ Bike

WORKED THESE ASSETS

- ◯ Chest
- ◯ Shoulders

- ◯ Back
- ◯ Arms

- ◯ Legs
- ◯ Abs

How'd it go?   😍   🙂   😐   🙁   😵

Details: _____
_____
_____
_____
_____

BONUS MOVES

- ◯ Took the stairs
- ◯ Added steps
- ◯ Went for a walking meeting

- ◯ Walked the dog
- ◯ Went dancing with friends
- ◯ Other: _____

MOOD & ENERGY REPORT

_____
_____
_____
_____
_____
_____
_____

STRESS LEVEL

○ Fried
○ A mixed bag
○ Could vaguely imagine being calm

○ Cucumber cool
○ I own this town

This made me smile: _____

TODAY'S MENU FEATURED

BREAKFAST
_____
_____
_____

LUNCH
_____
_____
_____

DINNER
_____
_____
_____

SNACKS
_____
_____
_____

WATER _____ OZ

My most brilliant choice today: _____

I could use a do-over on this one: _____

I'll make tomorrow even more awesome by: _____

_____

_____

Date: _____ (S) (M) (T) (W) (Th) (F) (S)

WORKOUT

- ( ) Cardio
- ( ) Strength
- ( ) Yoga
- ( ) Other: _____
- ( ) Pilates
- ( ) Walk
- ( ) Swim
- ( ) Run
- ( ) Bike

WORKED THESE ASSETS

- ( ) Chest
- ( ) Shoulders
- ( ) Back
- ( ) Arms
- ( ) Legs
- ( ) Abs

How'd it go?   😍   🙂   😐   🙁   😵

Details: _____

_____

_____

_____

_____

BONUS MOVES

- ( ) Took the stairs
- ( ) Added steps
- ( ) Went for a walking meeting
- ( ) Walked the dog
- ( ) Went dancing with friends
- ( ) Other: _____

MOOD & ENERGY REPORT

_____

_____

_____

_____

_____

_____

_____

○ Fried
○ A mixed bag
○ Could vaguely imagine being calm

○ Cucumber cool
○ I own this town

This made me smile: _____

TODAY'S MENU FEATURED

BREAKFAST
_____
_____
_____

LUNCH
_____
_____
_____

DINNER
_____
_____
_____

SNACKS
_____
_____
_____

WATER _____ OZ

My most brilliant choice today: _____

I could use a do-over on this one: _____

I'll make tomorrow even more awesome by: _____

_____

_____

Date: _____   (S) (M) (T) (W) (Th) (F) (S)

WORKOUT

- ◯ Cardio   ◯ Pilates   ◯ Run
- ◯ Strength   ◯ Walk   ◯ Bike
- ◯ Yoga   ◯ Swim
- ◯ Other: _____

WORKED THESE ASSETS

- ◯ Chest   ◯ Back   ◯ Legs
- ◯ Shoulders   ◯ Arms   ◯ Abs

How'd it go?   😍   🙂   😐   🙁   😵

Details: _____
_____
_____
_____
_____

BONUS MOVES

- ◯ Took the stairs   ◯ Walked the dog
- ◯ Added steps   ◯ Went dancing with friends
- ◯ Went for a walking meeting ◯ Other: _____

MOOD & ENERGY REPORT

_____
_____
_____
_____
_____
_____
_____

STRESS LEVEL

○ Fried
○ A mixed bag
○ Could vaguely imagine
   being calm

○ Cucumber cool
○ I own this town

This made me smile: _____

TODAY'S MENU FEATURED

BREAKFAST
_____
_____
_____

LUNCH
_____
_____
_____

DINNER
_____
_____
_____

SNACKS
_____
_____
_____

WATER _____ OZ

My most brilliant choice today: _____

I could use a do-over on this one: _____

I'll make tomorrow even more awesome by: _____

_____
_____

Date: _____ (S) (M) (T) (W) (Th) (F) (S)

WORKOUT

- ◯ Cardio
- ◯ Strength
- ◯ Yoga
- ◯ Other: _____

- ◯ Pilates
- ◯ Walk
- ◯ Swim

- ◯ Run
- ◯ Bike

WORKED THESE ASSETS

- ◯ Chest
- ◯ Shoulders

- ◯ Back
- ◯ Arms

- ◯ Legs
- ◯ Abs

How'd it go?   😍   🙂   😐   🙁   😵

Details: _____

_____

_____

_____

_____

BONUS MOVES

- ◯ Took the stairs
- ◯ Added steps
- ◯ Went for a walking meeting

- ◯ Walked the dog
- ◯ Went dancing with friends
- ◯ Other: _____

MOOD & ENERGY REPORT

_____

_____

_____

_____

_____

_____

_____

○ Fried   ○ Cucumber cool
○ A mixed bag   ○ I own this town
○ Could vaguely imagine
   being calm

This made me smile: _____

TODAY'S MENU FEATURED

BREAKFAST
_____
_____
_____

LUNCH
_____
_____
_____

DINNER
_____
_____
_____

SNACKS
_____
_____
_____

WATER _____ OZ

My most brilliant choice today: _____

I could use a do-over on this one: _____

I'll make tomorrow even more awesome by: _____

_____

_____

Date: _____ ⓈⓂⓉⓌ(Th)ⒻⓈ

WORKOUT

- ◯ Cardio
- ◯ Strength
- ◯ Yoga
- ◯ Other: _____

- ◯ Pilates
- ◯ Walk
- ◯ Swim

- ◯ Run
- ◯ Bike

WORKED THESE ASSETS

- ◯ Chest
- ◯ Shoulders

- ◯ Back
- ◯ Arms

- ◯ Legs
- ◯ Abs

How'd it go?   😍   🙂   😐   🙁   😵

Details: _____

_____

_____

_____

_____

BONUS MOVES

- ◯ Took the stairs
- ◯ Added steps
- ◯ Went for a walking meeting

- ◯ Walked the dog
- ◯ Went dancing with friends
- ◯ Other: _____

MOOD & ENERGY REPORT

_____

_____

_____

_____

_____

_____

_____

○ Fried
○ A mixed bag
○ Could vaguely imagine being calm

○ Cucumber cool
○ I own this town

This made me smile: _____

TODAY'S MENU FEATURED

BREAKFAST
_____
_____
_____

LUNCH
_____
_____
_____

DINNER
_____
_____
_____

SNACKS
_____
_____
_____

WATER _____ OZ

My most brilliant choice today: _____

I could use a do-over on this one: _____

I'll make tomorrow even more awesome by: _____

_____

_____

Date: _____   (S) (M) (T) (W) (Th) (F) (S)

WORKOUT

- ◯ Cardio   ◯ Pilates   ◯ Run
- ◯ Strength   ◯ Walk   ◯ Bike
- ◯ Yoga   ◯ Swim
- ◯ Other: _____

WORKED THESE ASSETS

- ◯ Chest   ◯ Back   ◯ Legs
- ◯ Shoulders   ◯ Arms   ◯ Abs

How'd it go?   😍   🙂   😐   🙁   😵

Details: _____

_____

_____

_____

_____

BONUS MOVES

- ◯ Took the stairs   ◯ Walked the dog
- ◯ Added steps   ◯ Went dancing with friends
- ◯ Went for a walking meeting   ◯ Other: _____

MOOD & ENERGY REPORT

_____

_____

_____

_____

_____

_____

_____

STRESS LEVEL

- ◯ Fried
- ◯ A mixed bag
- ◯ Could vaguely imagine being calm
- ◯ Cucumber cool
- ◯ I own this town

This made me smile: _____

TODAY'S MENU FEATURED

BREAKFAST
_____
_____
_____

LUNCH
_____
_____
_____

DINNER
_____
_____
_____

SNACKS
_____
_____
_____

WATER _____ OZ

My most brilliant choice today: _____

I could use a do-over on this one: _____

I'll make tomorrow even more awesome by: _____

_____

_____

Date: _____ (S) (M) (T) (W) (Th) (F) (S)

WORKOUT

- ◯ Cardio
- ◯ Strength
- ◯ Yoga
- ◯ Other: _____

- ◯ Pilates
- ◯ Walk
- ◯ Swim

- ◯ Run
- ◯ Bike

WORKED THESE ASSETS

- ◯ Chest
- ◯ Shoulders

- ◯ Back
- ◯ Arms

- ◯ Legs
- ◯ Abs

How'd it go? 😍 🙂 😐 🙁 😵

Details: _____

_____

_____

_____

_____

BONUS MOVES

- ◯ Took the stairs
- ◯ Added steps
- ◯ Went for a walking meeting

- ◯ Walked the dog
- ◯ Went dancing with friends
- ◯ Other: _____

MOOD & ENERGY REPORT

_____

_____

_____

_____

_____

_____

_____

STRESS LEVEL

◯ Fried
◯ A mixed bag
◯ Could vaguely imagine being calm

◯ Cucumber cool
◯ I own this town

This made me smile: _____

TODAY'S MENU FEATURED

BREAKFAST
_____
_____
_____

LUNCH
_____
_____
_____

DINNER
_____
_____
_____

SNACKS
_____
_____
_____

WATER _____ OZ

My most brilliant choice today: _____

I could use a do-over on this one: _____

I'll make tomorrow even more awesome by: _____

_____

_____

Date: _____   (S) (M) (T) (W) (Th) (F) (S)

WORKOUT

- ◯ Cardio
- ◯ Strength
- ◯ Yoga
- ◯ Other: _____

- ◯ Pilates
- ◯ Walk
- ◯ Swim

- ◯ Run
- ◯ Bike

WORKED THESE ASSETS

- ◯ Chest
- ◯ Shoulders

- ◯ Back
- ◯ Arms

- ◯ Legs
- ◯ Abs

How'd it go?   😍   🙂   😐   🙁   😵

Details: _____
_____
_____
_____
_____

BONUS MOVES

- ◯ Took the stairs
- ◯ Added steps
- ◯ Went for a walking meeting

- ◯ Walked the dog
- ◯ Went dancing with friends
- ◯ Other: _____

MOOD & ENERGY REPORT

_____
_____
_____
_____
_____
_____
_____

STRESS LEVEL

◯ Fried
◯ A mixed bag
◯ Could vaguely imagine being calm

◯ Cucumber cool
◯ I own this town

This made me smile: _____

TODAY'S MENU FEATURED

BREAKFAST
_____
_____
_____

LUNCH
_____
_____
_____

DINNER
_____
_____
_____

SNACKS
_____
_____
_____

WATER _____ OZ

My most brilliant choice today: _____
I could use a do-over on this one: _____
I'll make tomorrow even more awesome by: _____
_____
_____

Date: _____ (S) (M) (T) (W) (Th) (F) (S)

WORKOUT

- ◯ Cardio
- ◯ Strength
- ◯ Yoga
- ◯ Other: _____

- ◯ Pilates
- ◯ Walk
- ◯ Swim

- ◯ Run
- ◯ Bike

WORKED THESE ASSETS

- ◯ Chest
- ◯ Shoulders

- ◯ Back
- ◯ Arms

- ◯ Legs
- ◯ Abs

How'd it go?   (😍)   (🙂)   (😐)   (🙁)   (😵)

Details: _____

_____

_____

_____

_____

BONUS MOVES

- ◯ Took the stairs
- ◯ Added steps
- ◯ Went for a walking meeting

- ◯ Walked the dog
- ◯ Went dancing with friends
- ◯ Other: _____

MOOD & ENERGY REPORT

_____

_____

_____

_____

_____

_____

_____

STRESS LEVEL

○ Fried
○ A mixed bag
○ Could vaguely imagine being calm

○ Cucumber cool
○ I own this town

This made me smile: _____

TODAY'S MENU FEATURED

BREAKFAST
_____
_____
_____

LUNCH
_____
_____
_____

DINNER
_____
_____
_____

SNACKS
_____
_____
_____

WATER _____ OZ

My most brilliant choice today: _____
I could use a do-over on this one: _____
I'll make tomorrow even more awesome by: _____
_____
_____

Date: _____ (S) (M) (T) (W) (Th) (F) (S)

WORKOUT

- ◯ Cardio   ◯ Pilates   ◯ Run
- ◯ Strength   ◯ Walk   ◯ Bike
- ◯ Yoga   ◯ Swim
- ◯ Other: _____

WORKED THESE ASSETS

- ◯ Chest   ◯ Back   ◯ Legs
- ◯ Shoulders   ◯ Arms   ◯ Abs

How'd it go?   😍   🙂   😐   🙁   😵

Details: _____
_____
_____
_____
_____

BONUS MOVES

- ◯ Took the stairs   ◯ Walked the dog
- ◯ Added steps   ◯ Went dancing with friends
- ◯ Went for a walking meeting   ◯ Other: _____

MOOD & ENERGY REPORT

_____
_____
_____
_____
_____
_____
_____

○ Fried
○ A mixed bag
○ Could vaguely imagine being calm

○ Cucumber cool
○ I own this town

This made me smile: _____

TODAY'S MENU FEATURED

BREAKFAST
_____
_____
_____

LUNCH
_____
_____
_____

DINNER
_____
_____
_____

SNACKS
_____
_____
_____

WATER _____ OZ

My most brilliant choice today: _____

I could use a do-over on this one: _____

I'll make tomorrow even more awesome by: _____

_____

_____

Date: _____ (S) (M) (T) (W) (Th) (F) (S)

WORKOUT

- ◯ Cardio
- ◯ Strength
- ◯ Yoga
- ◯ Other: _____

- ◯ Pilates
- ◯ Walk
- ◯ Swim

- ◯ Run
- ◯ Bike

WORKED THESE ASSETS

- ◯ Chest
- ◯ Shoulders

- ◯ Back
- ◯ Arms

- ◯ Legs
- ◯ Abs

How'd it go? 😍 🙂 😐 🙁 😵

Details: _____

_____

_____

_____

_____

BONUS MOVES

- ◯ Took the stairs
- ◯ Added steps
- ◯ Went for a walking meeting

- ◯ Walked the dog
- ◯ Went dancing with friends
- ◯ Other: _____

MOOD & ENERGY REPORT

_____

_____

_____

_____

_____

_____

_____

STRESS LEVEL

○ Fried
○ A mixed bag
○ Could vaguely imagine being calm

○ Cucumber cool
○ I own this town

This made me smile: _____

TODAY'S MENU FEATURED

BREAKFAST
_____
_____
_____

LUNCH
_____
_____
_____

DINNER
_____
_____
_____

SNACKS
_____
_____
_____

WATER _____ OZ

My most brilliant choice today: _____

I could use a do-over on this one: _____

I'll make tomorrow even more awesome by: _____

_____

_____

Date: _____   (S) (M) (T) (W) (Th) (F) (S)

WORKOUT

- ◯ Cardio
- ◯ Strength
- ◯ Yoga
- ◯ Other: _____

- ◯ Pilates
- ◯ Walk
- ◯ Swim

- ◯ Run
- ◯ Bike

WORKED THESE ASSETS

- ◯ Chest
- ◯ Shoulders

- ◯ Back
- ◯ Arms

- ◯ Legs
- ◯ Abs

How'd it go?   😍   🙂   😐   🙁   😵

Details: _____
_____
_____
_____
_____

BONUS MOVES

- ◯ Took the stairs
- ◯ Added steps
- ◯ Went for a walking meeting

- ◯ Walked the dog
- ◯ Went dancing with friends
- ◯ Other: _____

MOOD & ENERGY REPORT

_____
_____
_____
_____
_____
_____
_____

◯ Fried
◯ A mixed bag
◯ Could vaguely imagine
being calm

◯ Cucumber cool
◯ I own this town

This made me smile: _____

TODAY'S MENU FEATURED

BREAKFAST
_____
_____
_____

LUNCH
_____
_____
_____

DINNER
_____
_____
_____

SNACKS
_____
_____
_____

WATER _____ OZ

My most brilliant choice today: _____

I could use a do-over on this one: _____

I'll make tomorrow even more awesome by: _____

_____
_____

Date: _____ (S) (M) (T) (W) (Th) (F) (S)

WORKOUT

- ◯ Cardio
- ◯ Strength
- ◯ Yoga
- ◯ Other: _____

- ◯ Pilates
- ◯ Walk
- ◯ Swim

- ◯ Run
- ◯ Bike

WORKED THESE ASSETS

- ◯ Chest
- ◯ Shoulders

- ◯ Back
- ◯ Arms

- ◯ Legs
- ◯ Abs

How'd it go?   😍   🙂   😐   🙁   😵

Details: _____

_____

_____

_____

_____

BONUS MOVES

- ◯ Took the stairs
- ◯ Added steps
- ◯ Went for a walking meeting

- ◯ Walked the dog
- ◯ Went dancing with friends
- ◯ Other: _____

MOOD & ENERGY REPORT

_____

_____

_____

_____

_____

_____

_____

STRESS LEVEL

○ Fried
○ A mixed bag
○ Could vaguely imagine being calm

○ Cucumber cool
○ I own this town

This made me smile: _____

TODAY'S MENU FEATURED

BREAKFAST
_____
_____
_____

LUNCH
_____
_____
_____

DINNER
_____
_____
_____

SNACKS
_____
_____
_____

WATER _____ OZ

My most brilliant choice today: _____

I could use a do-over on this one: _____

I'll make tomorrow even more awesome by: _____

_____

_____

MAKE YOUR OWN RULES,

DON'T FOLLOW ANYONE ELSE'S.

Date: _____   (S) (M) (T) (W) (Th) (F) (S)

WORKOUT

○ Cardio   ○ Pilates   ○ Run
○ Strength   ○ Walk   ○ Bike
○ Yoga   ○ Swim
○ Other: _____

WORKED THESE ASSETS

○ Chest   ○ Back   ○ Legs
○ Shoulders   ○ Arms   ○ Abs

How'd it go?   😍   🙂   😐   🙁   😵

Details: _____

_____

_____

_____

_____

BONUS MOVES

○ Took the stairs   ○ Walked the dog
○ Added steps   ○ Went dancing with friends
○ Went for a walking meeting   ○ Other: _____

MOOD & ENERGY REPORT

_____

_____

_____

_____

_____

_____

_____

○ Fried   ○ Cucumber cool
○ A mixed bag   ○ I own this town
○ Could vaguely imagine
  being calm

This made me smile: _____

TODAY'S MENU FEATURED

BREAKFAST
_____
_____
_____

LUNCH
_____
_____
_____

DINNER
_____
_____
_____

SNACKS
_____
_____
_____

WATER _____ OZ

My most brilliant choice today: _____

I could use a do-over on this one: _____

I'll make tomorrow even more awesome by: _____

_____

_____

Date: _____ (S) (M) (T) (W) (Th) (F) (S)

WORKOUT

- ◯ Cardio
- ◯ Strength
- ◯ Yoga
- ◯ Other: _____

- ◯ Pilates
- ◯ Walk
- ◯ Swim

- ◯ Run
- ◯ Bike

WORKED THESE ASSETS

- ◯ Chest
- ◯ Shoulders

- ◯ Back
- ◯ Arms

- ◯ Legs
- ◯ Abs

How'd it go?   ☺   ☺   ☺   ☹   ☹

Details: _____

_____

_____

_____

_____

BONUS MOVES

- ◯ Took the stairs
- ◯ Added steps
- ◯ Went for a walking meeting

- ◯ Walked the dog
- ◯ Went dancing with friends
- ◯ Other: _____

MOOD & ENERGY REPORT

_____

_____

_____

_____

_____

_____

_____

○ Fried   ○ Cucumber cool
○ A mixed bag   ○ I own this town
○ Could vaguely imagine
  being calm

This made me smile: _____

TODAY'S MENU FEATURED

BREAKFAST
_____
_____
_____

LUNCH
_____
_____
_____

DINNER
_____
_____
_____

SNACKS
_____
_____
_____

WATER _____ OZ

My most brilliant choice today: _____

I could use a do-over on this one: _____

I'll make tomorrow even more awesome by: _____

_____

_____

Date: _____   (S) (M) (T) (W) (Th) (F) (S)

WORKOUT

- ◯ Cardio
- ◯ Strength
- ◯ Yoga
- ◯ Other: _____

- ◯ Pilates
- ◯ Walk
- ◯ Swim

- ◯ Run
- ◯ Bike

WORKED THESE ASSETS

- ◯ Chest
- ◯ Shoulders

- ◯ Back
- ◯ Arms

- ◯ Legs
- ◯ Abs

How'd it go?   😍   🙂   😐   🙁   😵

Details: _____

_____

_____

_____

_____

BONUS MOVES

- ◯ Took the stairs
- ◯ Added steps
- ◯ Went for a walking meeting

- ◯ Walked the dog
- ◯ Went dancing with friends
- ◯ Other: _____

MOOD & ENERGY REPORT

_____

_____

_____

_____

_____

_____

_____

STRESS LEVEL

◯ Fried
◯ A mixed bag
◯ Could vaguely imagine being calm

◯ Cucumber cool
◯ I own this town

This made me smile: _____

TODAY'S MENU FEATURED

BREAKFAST
_____
_____
_____

LUNCH
_____
_____
_____

DINNER
_____
_____
_____

SNACKS
_____
_____
_____

WATER _____ OZ

My most brilliant choice today: _____

I could use a do-over on this one: _____

I'll make tomorrow even more awesome by: _____

_____

_____

Date: _____   (S) (M) (T) (W) (Th) (F) (S)

WORKOUT

- ◯ Cardio
- ◯ Strength
- ◯ Yoga
- ◯ Other: _____

- ◯ Pilates
- ◯ Walk
- ◯ Swim

- ◯ Run
- ◯ Bike

WORKED THESE ASSETS

- ◯ Chest
- ◯ Shoulders

- ◯ Back
- ◯ Arms

- ◯ Legs
- ◯ Abs

How'd it go?   😍   🙂   😐   🙁   😫

Details: _____

_____

_____

_____

_____

BONUS MOVES

- ◯ Took the stairs
- ◯ Added steps
- ◯ Went for a walking meeting

- ◯ Walked the dog
- ◯ Went dancing with friends
- ◯ Other: _____

MOOD & ENERGY REPORT

_____

_____

_____

_____

_____

_____

_____

STRESS LEVEL

◯ Fried
◯ A mixed bag
◯ Could vaguely imagine
being calm

◯ Cucumber cool
◯ I own this town

This made me smile: _____

TODAY'S MENU FEATURED

BREAKFAST
_____
_____
_____

LUNCH
_____
_____
_____

DINNER
_____
_____
_____

SNACKS
_____
_____
_____

WATER _____ OZ

My most brilliant choice today: _____

I could use a do-over on this one: _____

I'll make tomorrow even more awesome by: _____

_____

_____

Date: _____ (S) (M) (T) (W) (Th) (F) (S)

WORKOUT

- ◯ Cardio
- ◯ Strength
- ◯ Yoga
- ◯ Other: _____

- ◯ Pilates
- ◯ Walk
- ◯ Swim

- ◯ Run
- ◯ Bike

WORKED THESE ASSETS

- ◯ Chest
- ◯ Shoulders

- ◯ Back
- ◯ Arms

- ◯ Legs
- ◯ Abs

How'd it go? 😍 🙂 😐 🙁 😣

Details: _____

_____

_____

_____

_____

BONUS MOVES

- ◯ Took the stairs
- ◯ Added steps
- ◯ Went for a walking meeting

- ◯ Walked the dog
- ◯ Went dancing with friends
- ◯ Other: _____

MOOD & ENERGY REPORT

_____

_____

_____

_____

_____

_____

_____

◯ Fried
◯ A mixed bag
◯ Could vaguely imagine being calm

◯ Cucumber cool
◯ I own this town

This made me smile: _____

TODAY'S MENU FEATURED

BREAKFAST
_____
_____
_____

LUNCH
_____
_____
_____

DINNER
_____
_____
_____

SNACKS
_____
_____
_____

WATER _____ OZ

My most brilliant choice today: _____

I could use a do-over on this one: _____

I'll make tomorrow even more awesome by: _____

_____

_____

Date: _____   (S) (M) (T) (W) (Th) (F) (S)

WORKOUT

- ○ Cardio
- ○ Strength
- ○ Yoga
- ○ Other: _____

- ○ Pilates
- ○ Walk
- ○ Swim

- ○ Run
- ○ Bike

WORKED THESE ASSETS

- ○ Chest
- ○ Shoulders

- ○ Back
- ○ Arms

- ○ Legs
- ○ Abs

How'd it go? 😍 🙂 😐 🙁 😵

Details: _____
_____
_____
_____
_____

BONUS MOVES

- ○ Took the stairs
- ○ Added steps
- ○ Went for a walking meeting

- ○ Walked the dog
- ○ Went dancing with friends
- ○ Other: _____

MOOD & ENERGY REPORT

_____
_____
_____
_____
_____
_____
_____

STRESS LEVEL

- ◯ Fried
- ◯ A mixed bag
- ◯ Could vaguely imagine being calm

- ◯ Cucumber cool
- ◯ I own this town

This made me smile: _____

TODAY'S MENU FEATURED

BREAKFAST
_____
_____
_____

LUNCH
_____
_____
_____

DINNER
_____
_____
_____

SNACKS
_____
_____
_____

WATER _____ OZ

My most brilliant choice today: _____

I could use a do-over on this one: _____

I'll make tomorrow even more awesome by: _____

_____

_____

Date: _____ (S) (M) (T) (W) (Th) (F) (S)

WORKOUT

- ◯ Cardio
- ◯ Strength
- ◯ Yoga
- ◯ Other: _____

- ◯ Pilates
- ◯ Walk
- ◯ Swim

- ◯ Run
- ◯ Bike

WORKED THESE ASSETS

- ◯ Chest
- ◯ Shoulders

- ◯ Back
- ◯ Arms

- ◯ Legs
- ◯ Abs

How'd it go? 😍 🙂 😐 🙁 😵

Details: _____

_____

_____

_____

_____

BONUS MOVES

- ◯ Took the stairs
- ◯ Added steps
- ◯ Went for a walking meeting

- ◯ Walked the dog
- ◯ Went dancing with friends
- ◯ Other: _____

MOOD & ENERGY REPORT

_____

_____

_____

_____

_____

_____

○ Fried
○ A mixed bag
○ Could vaguely imagine being calm

○ Cucumber cool
○ I own this town

This made me smile: _____

TODAY'S MENU FEATURED

BREAKFAST
_____
_____
_____

LUNCH
_____
_____
_____

DINNER
_____
_____
_____

SNACKS
_____
_____
_____

WATER _____ OZ

My most brilliant choice today: _____
I could use a do-over on this one: _____
I'll make tomorrow even more awesome by: _____
_____
_____

Date: _____ (S) (M) (T) (W) (Th) (F) (S)

WORKOUT

- ◯ Cardio
- ◯ Strength
- ◯ Yoga
- ◯ Other: _____

- ◯ Pilates
- ◯ Walk
- ◯ Swim

- ◯ Run
- ◯ Bike

WORKED THESE ASSETS

- ◯ Chest
- ◯ Shoulders

- ◯ Back
- ◯ Arms

- ◯ Legs
- ◯ Abs

How'd it go?   😍   🙂   😐   🙁   😵

Details: _____

_____

_____

_____

_____

BONUS MOVES

- ◯ Took the stairs
- ◯ Added steps
- ◯ Went for a walking meeting

- ◯ Walked the dog
- ◯ Went dancing with friends
- ◯ Other: _____

MOOD & ENERGY REPORT

_____

_____

_____

_____

_____

_____

_____

○ Fried   ○ Cucumber cool
○ A mixed bag   ○ I own this town
○ Could vaguely imagine
  being calm

This made me smile: _____

TODAY'S MENU FEATURED

BREAKFAST
_____
_____
_____

LUNCH
_____
_____
_____

DINNER
_____
_____
_____

SNACKS
_____
_____
_____

WATER _____ OZ

My most brilliant choice today: _____

I could use a do-over on this one: _____

I'll make tomorrow even more awesome by: _____

_____

_____

Date: _____ (S) (M) (T) (W) (Th) (F) (S)

WORKOUT

- ◯ Cardio
- ◯ Strength
- ◯ Yoga
- ◯ Other: _____

- ◯ Pilates
- ◯ Walk
- ◯ Swim

- ◯ Run
- ◯ Bike

WORKED THESE ASSETS

- ◯ Chest
- ◯ Shoulders

- ◯ Back
- ◯ Arms

- ◯ Legs
- ◯ Abs

How'd it go?   ☺   ☺   ☺   ☹   ☹

Details: _____

_____

_____

_____

_____

BONUS MOVES

- ◯ Took the stairs
- ◯ Added steps
- ◯ Went for a walking meeting

- ◯ Walked the dog
- ◯ Went dancing with friends
- ◯ Other: _____

MOOD & ENERGY REPORT

_____

_____

_____

_____

_____

_____

_____

◯ Fried
◯ A mixed bag
◯ Could vaguely imagine being calm

◯ Cucumber cool
◯ I own this town

This made me smile: _____

TODAY'S MENU FEATURED

BREAKFAST
_____
_____
_____

LUNCH
_____
_____
_____

DINNER
_____
_____
_____

SNACKS
_____
_____
_____

WATER _____ OZ

My most brilliant choice today: _____

I could use a do-over on this one: _____

I'll make tomorrow even more awesome by: _____

_____

_____

Date: _____   (S) (M) (T) (W) (Th) (F) (S)

WORKOUT

- ◯ Cardio
- ◯ Strength
- ◯ Yoga
- ◯ Other: _____

- ◯ Pilates
- ◯ Walk
- ◯ Swim

- ◯ Run
- ◯ Bike

WORKED THESE ASSETS

- ◯ Chest
- ◯ Shoulders

- ◯ Back
- ◯ Arms

- ◯ Legs
- ◯ Abs

How'd it go?   😍   🙂   😐   🙁   😵

Details: _____
_____
_____
_____
_____

BONUS MOVES

- ◯ Took the stairs
- ◯ Added steps
- ◯ Went for a walking meeting

- ◯ Walked the dog
- ◯ Went dancing with friends
- ◯ Other: _____

MOOD & ENERGY REPORT

_____
_____
_____
_____
_____
_____

STRESS LEVEL

○ Fried
○ A mixed bag
○ Could vaguely imagine being calm

○ Cucumber cool
○ I own this town

This made me smile: _____

TODAY'S MENU FEATURED

BREAKFAST
_____
_____
_____

LUNCH
_____
_____
_____

DINNER
_____
_____
_____

SNACKS
_____
_____
_____

WATER _____ OZ

My most brilliant choice today: _____
I could use a do-over on this one: _____
I'll make tomorrow even more awesome by: _____
_____
_____

Date: _____ (S) (M) (T) (W) (Th) (F) (S)

WORKOUT

- ◯ Cardio
- ◯ Strength
- ◯ Yoga
- ◯ Other: _____

- ◯ Pilates
- ◯ Walk
- ◯ Swim

- ◯ Run
- ◯ Bike

WORKED THESE ASSETS

- ◯ Chest
- ◯ Shoulders

- ◯ Back
- ◯ Arms

- ◯ Legs
- ◯ Abs

How'd it go?   😍   🙂   😐   🙁   😵

Details: _____

_____

_____

_____

_____

BONUS MOVES

- ◯ Took the stairs
- ◯ Added steps
- ◯ Went for a walking meeting

- ◯ Walked the dog
- ◯ Went dancing with friends
- ◯ Other: _____

MOOD & ENERGY REPORT

_____

_____

_____

_____

_____

_____

_____

STRESS LEVEL

◯ Fried

◯ A mixed bag

◯ Could vaguely imagine
being calm

◯ Cucumber cool

◯ I own this town

This made me smile: _____

TODAY'S MENU FEATURED

BREAKFAST
_____
_____
_____

LUNCH
_____
_____
_____

DINNER
_____
_____
_____

SNACKS
_____
_____
_____

WATER _____ OZ

My most brilliant choice today: _____

I could use a do-over on this one: _____

I'll make tomorrow even more awesome by: _____

_____

_____

Date: _____ (S) (M) (T) (W) (Th) (F) (S)

WORKOUT

- ◯ Cardio
- ◯ Strength
- ◯ Yoga
- ◯ Other: _____

- ◯ Pilates
- ◯ Walk
- ◯ Swim

- ◯ Run
- ◯ Bike

WORKED THESE ASSETS

- ◯ Chest
- ◯ Shoulders

- ◯ Back
- ◯ Arms

- ◯ Legs
- ◯ Abs

How'd it go?   😍   🙂   😐   🙁   😵

Details: _____

_____

_____

_____

_____

BONUS MOVES

- ◯ Took the stairs
- ◯ Added steps
- ◯ Went for a walking meeting

- ◯ Walked the dog
- ◯ Went dancing with friends
- ◯ Other: _____

MOOD & ENERGY REPORT

_____

_____

_____

_____

_____

_____

_____

STRESS LEVEL

◯ Fried
◯ A mixed bag
◯ Could vaguely imagine
  being calm

◯ Cucumber cool
◯ I own this town

This made me smile: _____

TODAY'S MENU FEATURED

BREAKFAST
_____
_____
_____

LUNCH
_____
_____
_____

DINNER
_____
_____
_____

SNACKS
_____
_____
_____

WATER _____ OZ

My most brilliant choice today: _____

I could use a do-over on this one: _____

I'll make tomorrow even more awesome by: _____

_____

_____

Date: _____   (S) (M) (T) (W) (Th) (F) (S)

WORKOUT

- ◯ Cardio
- ◯ Strength
- ◯ Yoga
- ◯ Other: _____

- ◯ Pilates
- ◯ Walk
- ◯ Swim

- ◯ Run
- ◯ Bike

WORKED THESE ASSETS

- ◯ Chest
- ◯ Shoulders

- ◯ Back
- ◯ Arms

- ◯ Legs
- ◯ Abs

How'd it go?   😍   🙂   😐   🙁   😵

Details: _____

_____

_____

_____

_____

BONUS MOVES

- ◯ Took the stairs
- ◯ Added steps
- ◯ Went for a walking meeting

- ◯ Walked the dog
- ◯ Went dancing with friends
- ◯ Other: _____

MOOD & ENERGY REPORT

_____

_____

_____

_____

_____

_____

_____

STRESS LEVEL

- ⭕ Fried
- ⭕ A mixed bag
- ⭕ Could vaguely imagine being calm

- ⭕ Cucumber cool
- ⭕ I own this town

This made me smile: _____

TODAY'S MENU FEATURED

BREAKFAST
_____
_____
_____

LUNCH
_____
_____
_____

DINNER
_____
_____
_____

SNACKS
_____
_____
_____

WATER _____ OZ

My most brilliant choice today: _____

I could use a do-over on this one: _____

I'll make tomorrow even more awesome by: _____

_____

_____

Date: _____ (S) (M) (T) (W) (Th) (F) (S)

WORKOUT

- ◯ Cardio
- ◯ Strength
- ◯ Yoga
- ◯ Other: _____

- ◯ Pilates
- ◯ Walk
- ◯ Swim

- ◯ Run
- ◯ Bike

WORKED THESE ASSETS

- ◯ Chest
- ◯ Shoulders

- ◯ Back
- ◯ Arms

- ◯ Legs
- ◯ Abs

How'd it go? (☻) (☺) (☺) (☹) (☓)

Details: _____
_____
_____
_____
_____

BONUS MOVES

- ◯ Took the stairs
- ◯ Added steps
- ◯ Went for a walking meeting

- ◯ Walked the dog
- ◯ Went dancing with friends
- ◯ Other: _____

MOOD & ENERGY REPORT

_____
_____
_____
_____
_____
_____
_____

STRESS LEVEL

- ○ Fried
- ○ A mixed bag
- ○ Could vaguely imagine being calm

- ○ Cucumber cool
- ○ I own this town

This made me smile: _____

TODAY'S MENU FEATURED

BREAKFAST
_____
_____
_____

LUNCH
_____
_____
_____

DINNER
_____
_____
_____

SNACKS
_____
_____
_____

WATER _____ OZ

My most brilliant choice today: _____

I could use a do-over on this one: _____

I'll make tomorrow even more awesome by: _____

_____

_____

Date: _____   (S) (M) (T) (W) (Th) (F) (S)

WORKOUT

- ◯ Cardio
- ◯ Strength
- ◯ Yoga
- ◯ Other: _____

- ◯ Pilates
- ◯ Walk
- ◯ Swim

- ◯ Run
- ◯ Bike

WORKED THESE ASSETS

- ◯ Chest
- ◯ Shoulders

- ◯ Back
- ◯ Arms

- ◯ Legs
- ◯ Abs

How'd it go?   😍   🙂   😐   🙁   😵

Details: _____
_____
_____
_____
_____

BONUS MOVES

- ◯ Took the stairs
- ◯ Added steps
- ◯ Went for a walking meeting

- ◯ Walked the dog
- ◯ Went dancing with friends
- ◯ Other: _____

MOOD & ENERGY REPORT

_____
_____
_____
_____
_____
_____
_____

STRESS LEVEL

- ◯ Fried
- ◯ A mixed bag
- ◯ Could vaguely imagine being calm

- ◯ Cucumber cool
- ◯ I own this town

This made me smile: _____

TODAY'S MENU FEATURED

BREAKFAST
_____
_____
_____

LUNCH
_____
_____
_____

DINNER
_____
_____
_____

SNACKS
_____
_____
_____

WATER _____ OZ

My most brilliant choice today: _____

I could use a do-over on this one: _____

I'll make tomorrow even more awesome by: _____

_____

_____

ABOUT THE ILLUSTRATOR

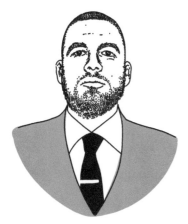

JESSE HORA's work never strays far from the ridiculous and playful while remaining detailed and incredibly thoughtful. His versatile skill set has lead him to become commercially successful, working with a wide range of clients, from international brands to local businesses to an up and coming gallery artist. Jesse has worked as a graphic designer and illustrator for 13 years, including for Adidas, Instagram, ESPN, Shake Shack, Herman Miller, and more. His *Food That Loves You Back* mural design for Roti can be seen at locations across the country. In 2011 he partnered with his lovely wife, Abby Wynne, to launch Make & Co, an artful creative company specializing in branding, graphic design, and mural design. Check out more of his work at jessehora.com and makeandco.com.

For general information on our other products and services or to obtain technical support, please contact our Customer Care Department within the United States at (866) 744-2665, or outside the United States at (510) 253-0500.

Rockridge Press publishes its books in a variety of electronic and print formats. Some content that appears in print may not be available in electronic books, and vice versa.

TRADEMARKS: Rockridge Press and the Rockridge Press logo are trademarks or registered trademarks of Callisto Media Inc. and/or its affiliates, in the United States and other countries, and may not be used without written permission. All other trademarks are the property of their respective owners. Rockridge Press is not associated with any product or vendor mentioned in this book.

Interior and Cover Designer: Heather Krakora
Art Producer: Tom Hood
Editor: Natasha Yglesias
Production Manager: Riley Hoffman
Production Editor: Sigi Nacson
Illustrations © Jesse Hora, 2020

ISBN: Print 978-1-64611-805-2

R0